Medical Food Book with Recipes

Life-Changing Foods for Your Healthy Life! Hidden Healing Powers of Smart and Super Foods.

(Best Medical Foods for Brain Health, for Heart Health, for Liver Health, for Thyroid Health, for Weight Loss)

By

Viktoria McCartney

Text Copyright [Viktoria McCartney]

Legal & Disclaimer

The information contained in this book and its contents is not designed to replace or take the place of any form of medical or professional advice; and is not meant to replace the need for independent medical, financial, legal, or other professional advice or services, as may be required. The content and information in this book have been provided for educational and entertainment purposes only.

The content and information contained in this book have been compiled from sources deemed reliable, and it is accurate to the best of the Author's knowledge, information, and belief. However, the Author cannot guarantee its accuracy and validity and cannot be held liable for any errors and/or omissions. Further, changes are periodically made to this book as and when needed. Where appropriate and/or necessary, you must consult a professional (including but not limited to your doctor, attorney, financial advisor or such other professional advisor) before using any of the suggested remedies, techniques, or information in this book.

Upon using the contents and information contained in this book, you agree to hold harmless the Author from and against any damages, costs, and expenses, including any legal fees potentially resulting from the application of any of the information provided by this book. This disclaimer applies to any of the loss, damages or injury caused by the use and application, whether directly or indirectly, of any advice or information presented, whether for breach of contract, tort, negligence, personal injury, criminal intent, or under any other cause of action.

You agree to accept all risks of using the information presented in this book.

You agree that, by continuing to read this book, where appropriate and/or necessary, you shall consult a professional (including but not limited to your doctor, attorney, or financial advisor or such other advisor as needed) before using any of the suggested remedies, techniques, or information in this book.

TABLE OF CONTENT

INTRODUCTION

Tibetian traditional medicine is one of the most ancient cultural healing modalities and one of the strongest out there. It utilizes modification to the diet, behavioural habit changes and therapy from nature to bring about healing effects.

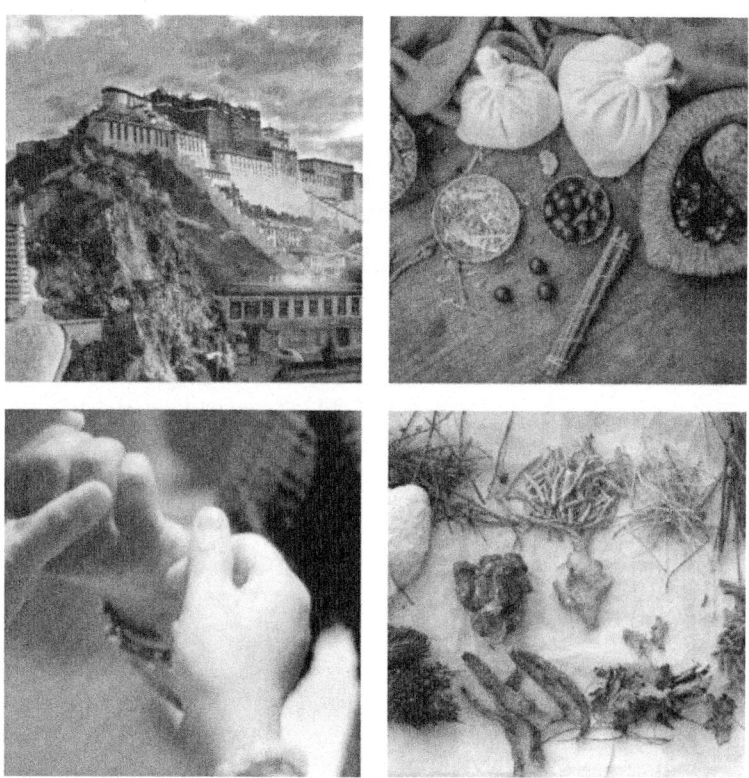

It originates from the Indian Buddhist beliefs in the concept that the illness stems from ignorance, aversion and attachment. For example, ignorance of which food items are poisonous and which are beneficial, attachment to unhealthy junk food and aversion towards unhealthy options.

The Tibetan traditional system is as ancient as the fifth century, yet information has effectively been passed from one generation to another and preserved over the centuries in the teachings of the four tantras.

The essence of Tibetan traditional medicine is to prevent illnesses and cure illnesses or imbalances. They use precise techniques to diagnose. The cultural teachings of the medicine entail the importance of balance between the different body systems and the connection between the diet and the health of different organs.

Knowledge can fight illnesses and prevention can protect against the onset of diseases. This book is based on the Tibetan traditional basis of how a proper diet and strengthening our bodies with certain super foods can help prevent certain illness and protect our organs and organ systems.

In this book, I discuss various powerful super foods that can supercharge your health and protect your organ systems. I will share with you the most precious super foods targeted to each organ system.

HOW SUPER FOODS CAN HEAL YOUR BODY AND PROMOTE YOUR HEALTH

You are what you eat. That is because each thing you eat gets broken down and your body absorbs the minerals, vitamins and other compounds and divides it among your cells. Therefore, it is important that you make sure that you ingest the food that provides your body with the most useful compounds and healthy nutrients. There are tons of natural compounds out there, including vitamins, minerals, antioxidants, phytochemicals etc. Each of these chemicals has a function that assists your body cells.

The best thing you can do is to include superfoods in your diet. Superfoods are power foods that contain a great quantity of healthy nutrients and beneficial natural compounds like vitamins, minerals, antioxidants, etc. Super foods help you feel better, stronger and healthier as they provide your body cells with their micro needs to supercharge their healing and regeneration. Not only that, but super foods help protect your body against chronic illnesses and diseases of age and degeneration and even cancer!

When you incorporate super foods to your diet, you can take your health to the next level, boost your energy levels and ward off chronic illnesses. Keep reading to find out what are some of the best super foods for boosting the health of each organ system, including your skin, your liver, heart, brain and much more!

Best Super Food for the Brain

A key vital organ in your body is your brain. It consciously and subconsciously controls every life process in your body via complex neural pathways. The brain also has the centers for motor movement, memory, learning, emotional regulation and sensory perception. Because the brain controls and regulates so many of our conscious and unconscious activities, it utilises about 20% of the body's entire calorie needs. This emphasises the importance of the fuel (food) you provide your brain with.

You don't only need to provide your brain with energy loaded food that meets its intensive demands, but you also need to provide it with specific nutrients that optimise the brain health on the cellular and neural level. For example, Omega 3 fatty acids are the brain's best friend as they aid in building and repairing your brain cells, thus fighting against ageing and pathologic neurodegeneration such as Alzheimer's.

Taking care of the food you nourish your brain with is critical to your brain health on the short term and therefore your entire body functions and mental health and sharpness in the long term.

1. Oily Fish

It is common knowledge that oily fish are a great booster of brain health. That is because they contain high but safe concentrations of Omega 3 fatty acids. Many people vaguely understand that omega 3 fatty acids are great for brain health. There is truly a connection between boosted brain functions and high levels of Omega 3 fatty acids. However, let's look deeper into the science behind why omega 3 fatty acids are great for your brain structure and function.

Examples of oily fish include: Tuna, Salmon, Sardines, Salmon, Herring and Mackerel.

Why Omega 3 is your Brain's Best Friend

Omega 3 fatty acids are constituents of the protective membranes around the brain cells known as neurons. Defective neurons are the basis of many brain diseases and neuropathology, including multiple sclerosis. Unprotected neurons eventually result in neuronal damage which leads to disability and loss of function depending on the affected neurons and the extent of the damage. However, effectively protected neurons mean healthier brain cells, faster brain connections and therefore, enhanced cognitive function and thinking abilities. A study revealed that those with high levels of Omega 3 fatty acids displayed increased blood flow to their brain which meant their brains were provided with oxygen and nutrients at a faster rate than those with low Omega 3 fatty acids levels.

A study revealed that the cerebral cortex of the brain (the part responsible for many of the conscious functions such as learning, conscious thinking, behavior and motor and sensory functions) contains Docosahexaenoic acid (DHA) as its constituent. DHA is a type of Omega 3 fatty acid found in oily fish. This shows the link between Omega 3 fatty acids and improved cognitive functions, learning abilities, behavioral problems and even ADHD. Other studies claimed that regular consumption of Omega 3 fatty acids resulted in decreased risk of dementia and psychosis and fewer seizures in patients who have epilepsy.

2. Dark Chocolate:

If you love chocolate, you will be pleased to know that Dark chocolate is on the list of brain boosting food. This is due to its main ingredient, Cacao which has flavonoids, a powerful type of antioxidant.

Why are antioxidants important for your brain health?

All cells are sensitive to oxidative stress; however, among all cells, brain cells are the most sensitive and more critical when it comes to injury from oxidative stress. Oxidative stress in simple words results from various harmful molecules called free radicals that are very toxic to the cells. They pose an oxidizing kind of stress on your cells and require an antioxidant to neutralize their effects.

When there is oxidative stress, and you don't include food rich in antioxidants in your diet, your cells suffer as a result and receive a great deal of damage that accumulates over time. In the brain, the injury to the brain cells results in a decline of function and cognitive decline brain disease.

In addition to their antioxidant effects, the flavonoids in cacao support the neuronal and blood vessel growth in regions of the brain responsible for learning and memory. This stimulation of growth and blood flow consequently results in improved function, specifically, an enhancement in the memory and learning abilities.

3. **Berries**

Similar to dark chocolate, berries also contain the flavonoid antioxidant substance which protects your brain from damage. Research conducted supports that berries are brain-friendly foods that you can utilize and yield their benefits by adding them to your breakfast or snacks.

Berries are powerful as they contain several antioxidants such as caffeic acid, catechin, anthocyanin and quercetin. They help reduce the oxidative stress in your body and reduce inflammation. Chronic inflammation, such as that associated with joint diseases, negatively affects the brain and interferes with its neuronal healthy signalling mechanism. The substances in berries also help boost the brain plasticity which improves the brain cell to cell communication. In the long term, this results in enhanced cognitive functions and boosted learning and memorizing abilities. The antioxidant effects also delay age-related neuronal degeneration or cognitive decline.

Examples of Berries (Fruit, Drupe) include Blackberries, blueberries, strawberries, mulberries, blackcurrants, and cherries.

4. Oats

They are known as the grain for the brain due to their richness in vitamins and minerals such as vitamin B, E and potassium and zinc. This super food boosts the brain cognitive and memory function via its dual benefit of energy-boosting carbohydrates and the vitamins and minerals. It also helps to stimulate the release of serotonin in the brain which boosts feelings of general well being and happiness. A brain deficient in serotonin is the basis of many brain diseases.

5. Apples

You can boost your brain power with this superfood that keeps doctors away. It is rich in powerful antioxidants which protects your brain cells and preserves its functions. Studies show that eating apples is linked to improved brain health and the reduction and delay of onset of degenerative brain diseases such as Parkinson's or Alzheimers. The high amounts of acetylcholine boosted by apples help improve the brain's health.

6. Beans

These low glycemic index superfoods are slowly digested to provide a sustainable source of glucose for the brain. The main fuel for the brain is glucose. It is also rich in magnesium, zinc and even folate which help boost the brain health and improve neural signalling. It also contains vitamin B which improves neural cell communications.

7. Broccoli

Because of its high levels of vitamins, it has been known that broccoli can help prevent degenerative diseases such as Alzheimer's. It also contains choline which helps boost your memory functions and enhance your thinking abilities. It is also known to boost mood, especially in older people.

8. Avocado

You didn't know that each time you were eating guacamole or any avocado-based recipe you were doing your brain a huge favour. It is rich in many minerals and vitamins such as vitamin C, E and B. It helps boosts your memory, cognitive function and concentration levels. During exams, Avocados are the perfect superfood to eat to be smarter and more focused.

9. Egg Yolk

You can enjoy a healthy breakfast while boosting your brain health with egg yolk. This is one of the most concentrated sources of choline. This boosts cell signalling and neural connections. Studies have shown a link between eating egg yolks and improved memory and cognitive functions. It also has a crucial role in the brain development of fetuses.

10. Green Tea

Included just one cup of green tea to your daily diet can do miracles to your brain health. It has polyphenols and flavonoids which are powerful antioxidants that help shield your brain from toxic effects, ageing and early diseases. Studies show that drinking green tea is also associated with improved memory functions.

Top Super food Recipes for the Brain

❧

FROZEN BERRY YOGHURT

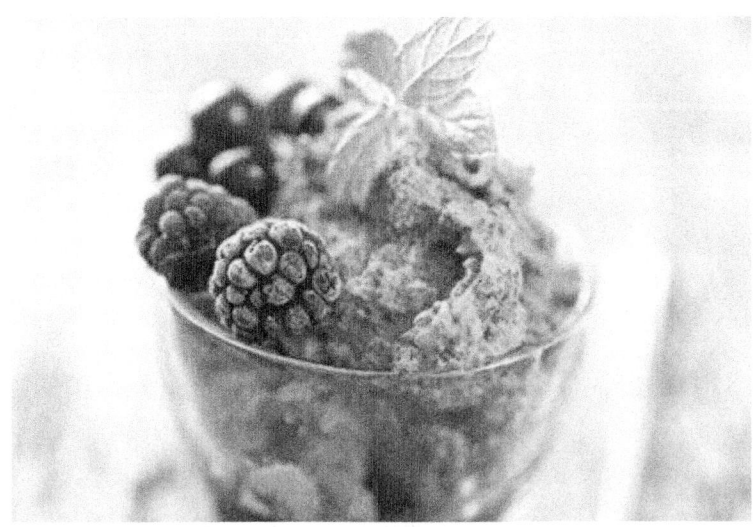

Total Prep Time: 10 Minutes

Yield: 2 Servings

INGREDIENTS

- 2 cups frozen mixed berries, divided
- 1 cup vanilla low-fat frozen yoghurt, divided
- 1/4 cup fat-free milk
- 1 tablespoon chopped fresh mint
- 1 tablespoon agave syrup

INSTRUCTIONS

1. Mix 1 cup of berries with 3/4 cup yoghurt and add the milk, mint, and agave syrup in food processor

2. Pulse until smooth.

3. Transfer into a freezer-safe container.

4. Add the remaining one cup of berries and the remaining 1/4 cup yoghurt to the processor; again, pulse until smooth.

5. Drip and swirl the berry mixture into the yogurt mixture.

6. Serve immediately or freeze until firm.

NUTRITIONAL INFORMATION

Calories 150

Fat 2.5g

Sat. fat 1.3g

Protein 6g

Carbohydrate 29g

Sugar 13 g

Fiber 2g

Cholesterol 33mg

Sodium 34mg

Calcium 155mg

BAKED SALMON

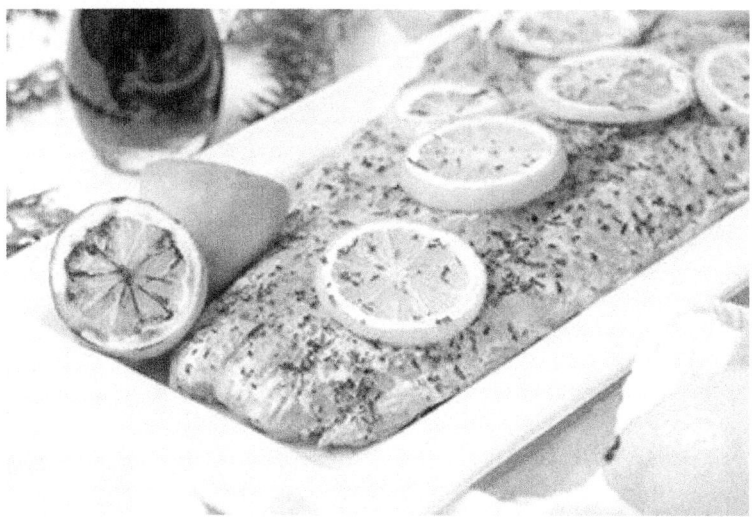

Total Prep Time: 35 Minutes

Yield: 4 Servings

INGREDIENTS

- 2 pounds salmon, I used Atlantic salmon
- 2 Tablespoons olive oil
- 3 garlic cloves, minced
- ¼ cup brown sugar

- ¼ cup soy sauce
- ½ teaspoon pepper
- juice of one lemon
- 1 teaspoon salt
- Sliced lemons and chopped parsley for garnish

INSTRUCTIONS

1. Preheat the oven to 350 degrees.
2. Use a baking pan and line it with aluminum foil. Place the salmon on top and sprinkle with salt and pepper to season.
3. Fold the aluminum foil around the salmon fish.
4. In a suitable sized bowl, mix together the olive oil, soy sauce, garlic, brown sugar, lemon juice, salt, and pepper.
5. Pour the prepared seasoning liquid glaze over the salmon and seal the aluminum foil.
6. Bake the salmon for 20-25 minutes.
7. Dip the salmon in the remaining sauce.
8. Garnish it with lemon slices and chopped parsley if desired.

NUTRITIONAL INFORMATION

Calories 280

Fat 3.1

Carbohydrates 13 G

Sugar 6g

Fiber 3g

Protein 12 G

 Cholesterol 0 Mg

Sodium 119 Mg

Calcium 4.2 %

AVOCADO EGG NESTS

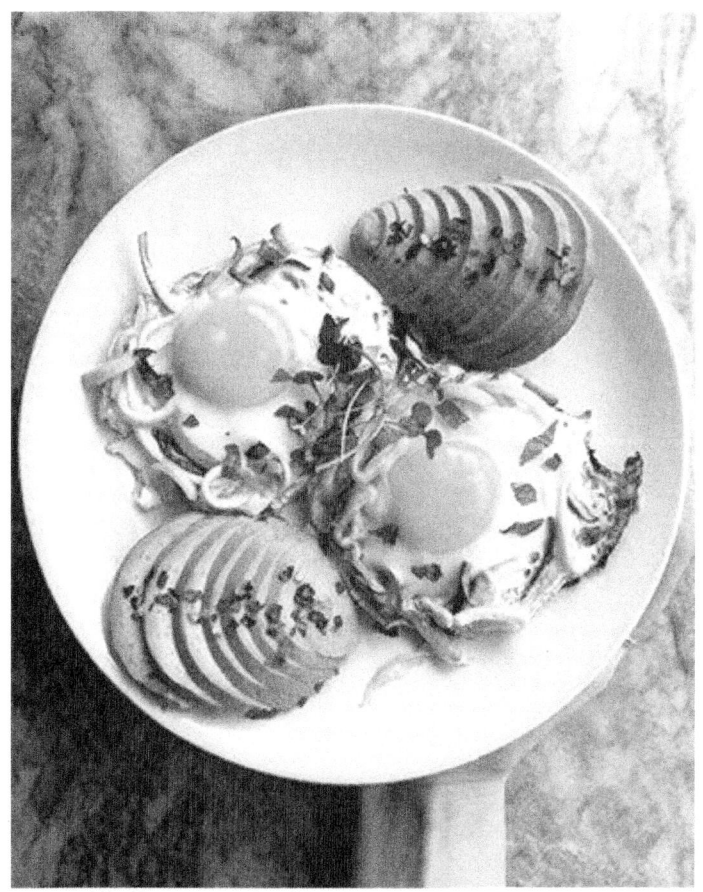

Total Prep Time: 20 Minutes

Yield: 4 Serving

INGREDIENTS

- 3 zucchinis, spiralized into noodles
- 2 tablespoons extra-virgin olive oil
- 4 large eggs
- Kosher salt and freshly ground black pepper
- 2 avocados, halved and thinly sliced
- Red-pepper flakes, for garnishing
- Fresh basil, for garnishing.

INSTRUCTIONS

1. Lightly grease a suitable baking sheet and Preheat the oven to 350°F.
2. In a suitable bowl, combine the zucchini noodles with olive oil and season with salt and pepper to taste.
3. Divide the noodles into 4 equal portions.
4. Move to the baking sheet and shape each bundle into a nest.
5. Crack an egg in the center of each avocado nest.
6. Bake for 9 to 11 minutes.
7. Season with salt and pepper to taste.
8. You can garnish with any choice such as red-pepper flakes and basil.
9. Serve with the baked avocado slices.

NUTRITIONAL INFORMATION

Calories 633

Total Fat 53g

Saturated 3 G

Carbohydrates 27g

Protein 20g

Sugars 9g

Fiber 10 G

Sodium 113 Mg

Calcium 8%

SUPER GREEN TEA SMOOTHIE

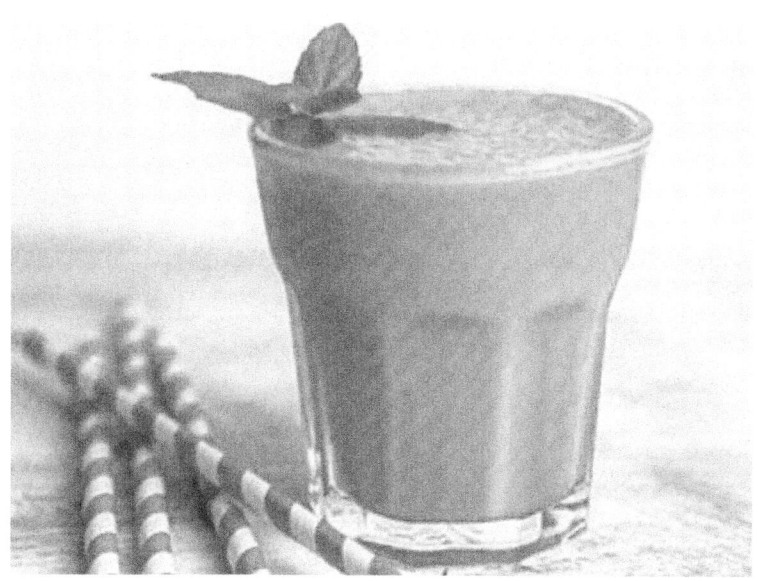

Total Prep Time: 10 Minutes

Yield: 1 Servings

INGREDIENTS

- 1 cup brewed green tea chilled
- 1 cup fresh spinach leaves
- 1 kiwi, peeled
- 1/4 avocado

- 1 banana, broken into chunks and frozen
- 1/2 teaspoon grated fresh ginger

INSTRUCTIONS

1. Add the tea, spinach, kiwi, banana, avocado, and ginger in a blender.
2. Blend until you get a smooth liquid.

NUTRITIONAL INFORMATION

Calories 120

Total fat 4.1 g

Saturated 0

Carbohydrates 22 g

Sugar 6 g

Fiber 2

Protein 2g

Cholesterol 0 mg

Sodium 19 mg

DARK CHOCOLATE CAKE

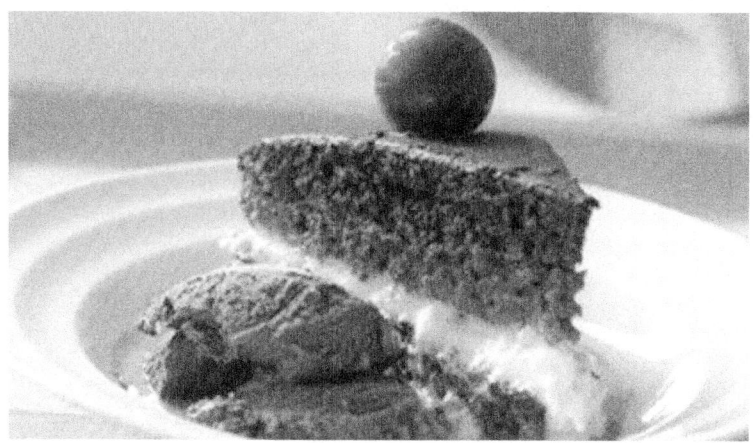

Total Prep Time: 40 Minutes

Yield: 12 Servings

INGREDIENTS

- 2 cups boiling water
- 1 cup unsweetened cocoa powder
- 2 3/4 cups all-purpose flour
- 2 teaspoons baking soda
- 1/2 teaspoon baking powder
- 1/2 teaspoon salt

- 1 cup butter, softened
- 2 1/4 cups white sugar
- 4 eggs
- 1 1/2 teaspoons vanilla extract

INSTRUCTIONS

1. Let the oven heat to 350 degrees F and prepare 3 - 9 inch round cake pans by greasing them.
2. In a suitable bowl, pour boiling water to the cocoa and whisk it until you get a smooth mixture.
3. In another medium bowl, add the flour, baking powder, baking soda, and salt and set it aside.
4. In another large bowl, add the cream butter and sugar whisk together until you get a light and fluffy texture.
5. Beat in the eggs one by one, next, add the vanilla.
6. Combine the flour mixture alternately with the cocoa mixture to the large bowl and whisk to get an even batter.
7. Spread the batter equally between the three greased pans.
8. Bake in the preheated oven for 25 to 30 minutes
9. Allow it to cool; you may decorate as desired.

NUTRITIONAL INFORMATION

Calories 427

Fat 18.3

Carbohydrates 63.8

Sugar 43 g

Fiber 10 g

Protein 6.6

Cholesterol 103

Sodium 465

APPLE SNICKERS SALAD

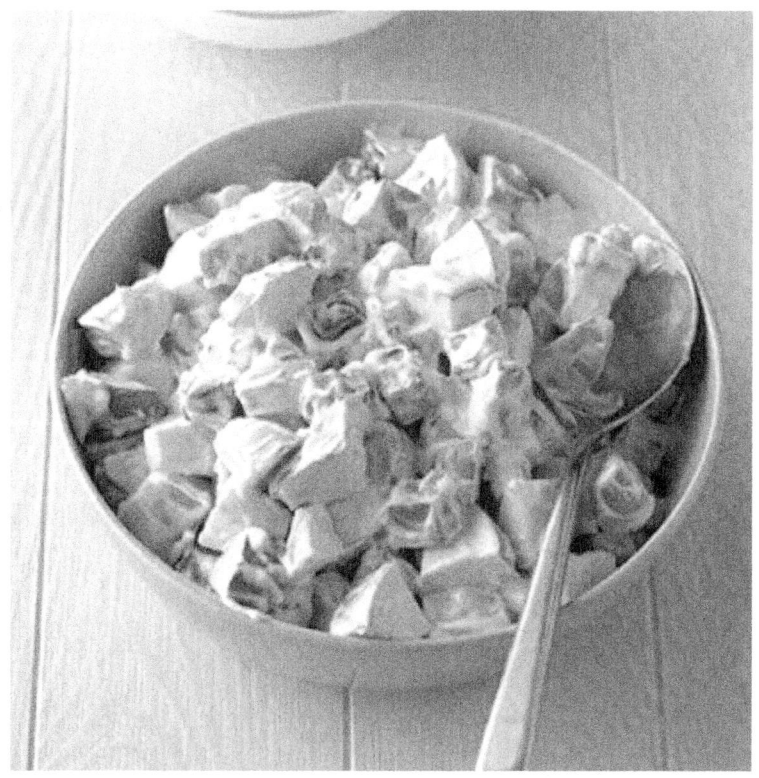

Total Prep Time: 5 Minutes

Yield: 4 Servings

INGREDIENTS

- 4 large green apples
- ½ cup milk
- caramel
- 2 snickers bars
- 8 oz whip cream
- 1 instant vanilla pudding

INSTRUCTIONS

1. Cut up apples and snickers and mix in.
2. Mix milk and vanilla pudding, pour it to the apples and garnish caramel.
3. Serve cold.

NUTRITIONAL INFORMATION

Calorie 2160

Fat: 89g

Carbohydrates 323g

Sodium 775 mg

Cholesterol 46 mg

Protein 30g

OAT MEAL PORRIDGE

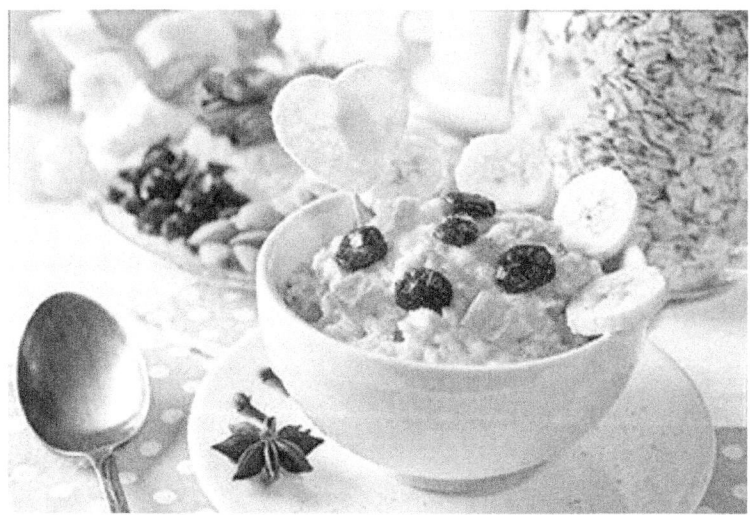

Total Prep Time: 30 Minutes

Yield: 4 Servings

INGREDIENTS

- 1-litre water
- 1 cup Oatmeal
- Sugar, Milk or cream, Black grapes for garnishing
- Salt to taste

INSTRUCTIONS

1. In a saucepan, take water to boil.

2. Pour the oatmeal into the boiling water, stir it continuously to prevent any lumps.

3. Add the salt and reduce the heat to low for 30 minutes, stir occasionally.

4. Serve with grapes, sugar and milk or cream.

NUTRITIONAL INFORMATION

Calorie: 117

Carbohydrates: 66.3 g

Sugar: 36 g

Fat : 6.9g

Fiber: 10.6 g

Protein: 16.9 g

RED BEANS AND RICE

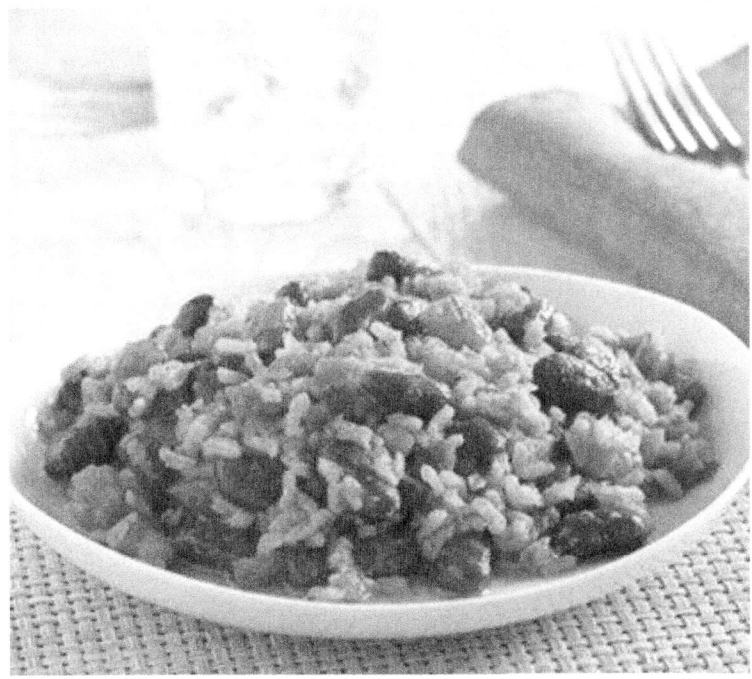

Total Prep Time: 60 Minutes

Yield: 4 Servings

INGREDIENTS

- 1 can kidney beans

- 4 ½ cups water
- 1 tablespoon olive oil
- 1 ½ cups tomato sauce
- ½ teaspoon dried oregano, dried basil
- Salt and pepper to taste
- 2 cups white rice (uncooked)
- 5 teaspoons adobo seasoning

INSTRUCTIONS

1. In a pan pour ½ cup water, oil, kidney beans, tomato sauce, oregano, basil, adobo.
2. Simmer on low heat for 25 mins or till the beans get boiled.
3. Serve hot beans over the rice.
4. On the other side, take 4 cups of water, boil it.
5. Then pour rice and stir. Simmer on low heat for 10 mins or till rice gets cooked. Add 3 teaspoons of adobo.

NUTRITIONAL INFORMATION

Calorie 511

Fat 5.1g

Sodium 710 mg

Carbohydrates 101g

Sugar 46 g

Fiber 32 g

Protein 14.5g

Calcium 8.2%

FRESH BROCCOLI SALAD

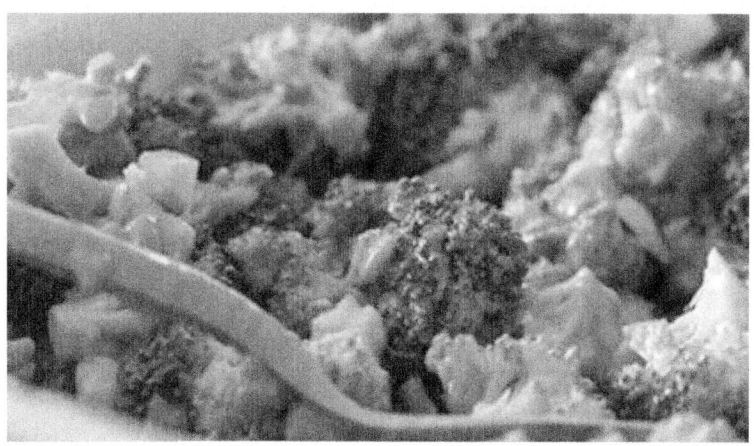

Total Prep Time: 30 Minutes

Yield: 4 Servings

INGREDIENTS

- 2 heads fresh broccoli
- 1 red onion
- 1/2 pound bacon
- 3/4 cup raisins
- 3/4 cup sliced almonds
- 1 cup mayonnaise

- 1/2 cup white sugar
- 2 tablespoons white wine vinegar

INSTRUCTIONS

1. Put the bacon in a deep skillet and let it cook over medium-high heat and crumble it after it cools.
2. Cut the broccoli into small pieces and chop the onion into thin bite-size slices.
3. Combine with the bacon, raisins, your favorite nuts and blend well.
4. To make the dressing, add the mayonnaise with the sugar and pour the vinegar together until smooth.
5. Stir the dressing into the salad, let chill and serve

NUTRITIONAL INFORMATION

Calories 374

Fat 27.2 g

Carbohydrates 28.5 g

Sugar 7 g

Fiber 18 g

Protein 7.3 g

Cholesterol 18 mg

Sodium 353 mg

DARK CHOCOLATE TRUFFLES

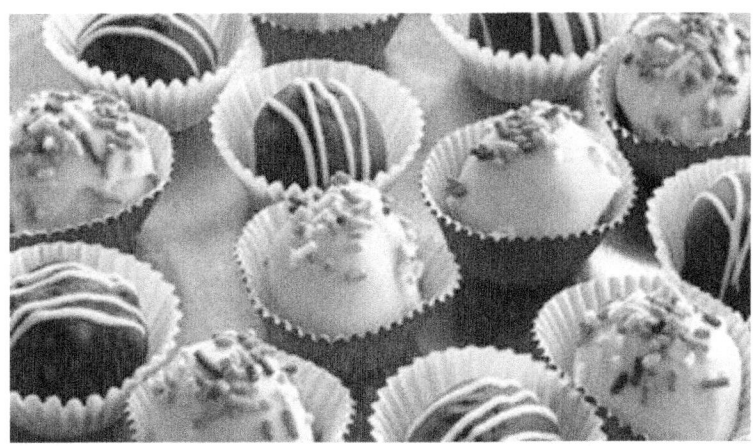

Total Prep Time: 10 Minutes

Yield: 4 Servings

INGREDIENTS

- 1 cup heavy cream
- 2 tablespoons butter
- 4 (1 ounce) squares baking chocolate
- 2 3/4 cups semi-sweet chocolate chips
- 2 tablespoons instant espresso powder (optional)

INSTRUCTIONS

1. Whisk the heavy cream with the butter, baking chocolate, chocolate chips, and the espresso powder in a saucepan over medium heat;

2. Let it cook till all your chocolate has melted into a smooth and thick mixture.

3. Remove it from the heat and transfer to a bowl and let it chill in refrigerator until the mixture hardens for around 1 hour.

4. Prepare a baking sheet then scoop small balls from the chocolate mixture onto the waxed paper. Store in refrigerator until the balls harden completely. Store in a cool, dry place.

NUTRITIONAL INFORMATION

Calories 87

Fat 7.1 g

Carbohydrates 6.8 g

Sugar 6.8 g

Fiber 0

Protein 1.2 g

Cholesterol 9 mg

Viktoria McCartney

Sodium 6 mg

Calcium 1%

BEST SUPER FOODS FOR HEART HEALTH

Aside from the fact that the heart is the source of all the love we feel, it's also an important organ in our body. It starts pumping from when we are in the womb before we are even born and until we die, it pumps nonstop and is the reason we continue to live because it supplies blood, oxygen and nutrients to all the parts of the body. That being the case, we need to take great care of it. Hence, here are some of the best foods that will help you maintain a healthy heart.

1. Oatmeal

Oatmeal is rich in soluble fibre. The fibre acts as a sponge in your body and absorbs fats, especially, cholesterol, thus lowering its levels and hence reducing its concentration in your bloodstream. When your cholesterol levels go unchecked, it will build up in various tissues in your body. The most dangerous spot is if it deposits in your arteries, especially the coronary arteries, a condition known as atherosclerosis which can eventually lead to ischemic heart disease (a heart disease where the heart does not have enough blood supply for itself) which is fatal.

You should also note that doctors recommend taking the old-fashioned oats instead of the instant oatmeal. That's because the instant oatmeal contains processed sugar which has its negative toll on your health as well.

2. Apples

You must have heard of the phrase, an apple a day keeps the doctor away. That is because apples can lower the risk of heart diseases. Apples contain phytochemicals known as Quercetin which will act as an anti-inflammatory agent. More to that, apples also have an antioxidant effect on the body. A constant inflammatory state reflects on your heart health; having a body free of inflammation reflects positively on your heart.

Apple's benefits are linked to the presence of polyphenols. One of the polyphenol compounds known as flavonoid epicatechin helps in lowering the blood pressure levels through promoting the relaxation of the arterial muscles. Increased blood pressure strains the heart and can result in heart failure over the long term. Lowered blood pressure helps take off the load from your heart so that you can prolong its health for as long as possible.

Like oatmeal, apples also have soluble fibre that is capable of absorbing cholesterol from the bloodstream. That reduces the chances of suffering from arteriosclerosis.

3. Olive oil

Olive oil is capable of reducing heart diseases by lowering cholesterol levels in the body. Contrary to popular belief, not all fats are harmful, some fats are actually healthy and reduce total cholesterol. Olive oil is an example of healthy, unsaturated fats. Also, diets rich in olive are able to reduce the damage on the endothelial cells which cover the inner surface of the blood vessels. The endothelial is a layer of cells in the arteries that helps with the blood flow, if the blood flow is flowing smoothly, the less the heart has to strain to compensate for the inefficiency of the arterial flow. Consider shifting from your regular cooking oil to cooking with olive oil

4. Avocados

Avocados are one of the most prominent heart-friendly foods. They help reduce the risk of developing heart diseases via various mechanisms, but the most important feature is that they decrease your blood cholesterol level and contains healthy fats. Avocados have a high concentration of monounsaturated fatty acid, which is considered a healthy type of fat that doesn't deposit on your arteries and clog them.

Avocados contain more potassium than bananas (bananas are known for being rich in potassium). The potassium helps your body to regulate its water content and reduces your blood pressure. Therefore, protecting your heart from heart failure related to hypertension.

Oleic acid which is one of the monounsaturated acids reduces the inflammation inside your body, especially your heart. They are rich in healthy nutrients while being low fat, that makes them an optimum option for nutritious food that provides energy and healthy nutrition without clogging the arteries. Moreover, they are rich in omega 3 which is a heart friendly fatty acid that promotes heart health.

5. Salmon

It is without doubt a popular knowledge that salmon is a very healthy addition to your daily diet. If you are aiming to protect and promote your heart health, eating salmon or any other oily fish can help reduce the risk of cardiac diseases by one third, which is a great percentage.

Oily fish like salmon are loaded with compounds like omega-3 fatty acids, DHA and EPA. DHA and EPA are known for reducing inflammation throughout the body, improving the functions of the epithelial cells and lowering blood pressure and protecting against blood clotting and thrombosis. These conditions pose huge risks to your cardiac health and your blood vessels which eventually drain into your heart. Any thrombosis could become a catastrophic health event; therefore, salmon and oily fish helps reduce the incidence of thrombosis and its predisposing factors.

Omega-3 also reduces inflammation throughout the body including the heart hence reducing risks of suffering from heart disease. While you can obtain omega 3 from supplements, studies have shown that it is the combination of all the other nutrients involved in the oily fish are what promote your heart health and protect it from diseases that you could be predisposed to. Salmon is known to boost your heart's health and reduce its risk of developing fatal heart diseases by a good percentage because it is one of the oily fish that contains omega 3 in a good percentage.

6. Tomatoes

There have been studies advocating for a tomato pill as it is known that the tomato can keep the doctor away and effectively reduce the risk of heart attacks. It contains potassium and lycopene. The lycopene acid which gives tomatoes its natural red colour is a powerful anti-oxidant which protects cells from becoming damaged.

Nutrients in tomatoes also help to lower the level of LDL and cholesterol which in turn helps to improve your lipid profile and protect your health from the effects of high levels of circulating fats, especially LDL. This lowers the risk of atherosclerosis and consequently the risk of strokes. It is also rich in folic acid, vitamin C and vitamin A.

Additionally, tomatoes have potassium which is a mineral that lowers blood pressure. This is done by taking away some of the sodium out of the body and relaxing the blood vessel walls. With the sodium out, you can decrease the volume load off your heart via the sodium-potassium dynamics.

Some studies suggested a correlation between the consumption of tomatoes and improved survival rates after heart attacks and patients of heart failure. The exact mechanism is not known but it could be due to the fact that tomatoes decrease inflammation and oxidative stress which decreases the quantity of damage on the heart. Also reducing the blood pressure reduces the load on a failing heart.

7. Liver

The liver has high levels of folic acid, chromium, iron, zinc, and copper which increase the levels of haemoglobin. Haemoglobin is the compound inside red blood cells that carries oxygen to our cells. Insufficient haemoglobin can lead to anaemia. Anaemia causes the heart to beat rapidly to compensate for the decrease blood oxygenation which strains the heart over time. Protect your heart by making sure you have all that you need to support your body cells and maintain sufficient oxygenation.

Moreover, liver is a nutritious food, that contains huge amounts of vitamin A which is anti-oxidant against cell damage by free radicals.

8. Asparagus

There are so many reasons you can add this super food to your diet. It is known for its cardio protective effects and its pressure reducing abilities. It helps flush your body of excess toxins. Asparagus helps prevent the build-up of homocysteine in the body. When there's a high level of homocysteine, you are likely to suffer from heart conditions which include stroke, among others.

It also aids your body to get rid of excess salts which can lower your blood pressure to healthy levels. If you have low coagulation, the vitamin K in asparagus can help you with coagulation. However, don't take excess asparagus if you have excess coagubility or a history of thrombosis as it can complicate the situation.

9. Berries

Berries are one of the most beneficial and delicious super foods. They contain a number of features which makes them friendly to your heart and reduce the risk of heart failure and strokes. They can help your blood flow smoothly and lower your lipid profile as they have zero saturated fats. Berries are packed with high levels of fibre which promote your heart health. They are a rich source of calcium, vitamin A and C, and polyphenols. These nutrients will help reduce any risk of heart failure. Also, berries are low on fat and have zero saturated fats which help reduce your overall weight, cholesterol levels and reduce your risk of heart diseases. Studies have proved the link between the consumption of berries and improved heart health. Be sure to pack some berries as a snack.

10. Nuts

Nuts such as almonds and pistachio are optimum for your heart health as they contain suitable amounts of healthy fats. They are full of minerals, fibre, antioxidants, and vitamins. Collectively, they help reduce the oxidative stress on your heart and provide it with healthy nutrients. They also have high levels of omega-3 which helps to reduce inflammation and in turn reduces risks of heart problems. They increase your HDL which shifts your lipid profile towards a healthy balance. What is more perfect than snacking while also protecting your heart from the risk of fatal diseases?

Top Super food Recipes for Heart Health

AVOCADO GLUCAMORE

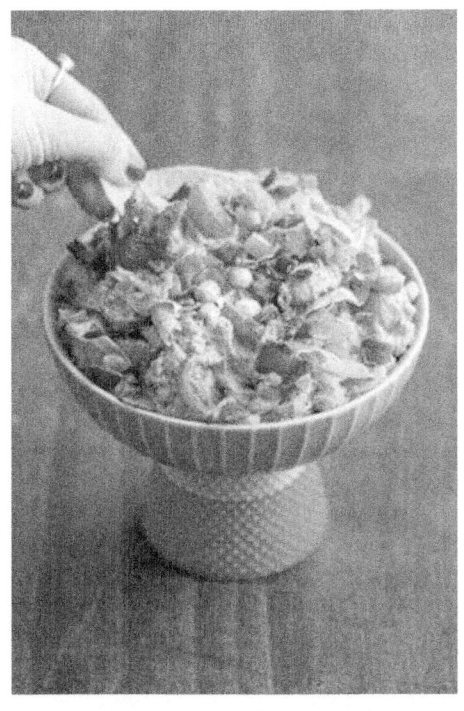

Total Prep Time: 15 minutes

Yields: 6 Servings

INGREDIENTS

- 2 mature avocados,
- ½ Cup Lettuce
- 1 Cup cherry tomatoes, halved
- 4 Slices of bacon, diced and cooked
- ¼ Cup green onions
- 2 Limes (Juice extract)
- 1 Tablespoon of kosher salt
- Freshly ground black pepper
- Tortilla chip may be added for serving if you desire

INSTRUCTIONS

1. Mash avocados in a large bowl
2. Add tomatoes, lettuce, green onions, and bacon and stir to mix. Squeeze and spread lime juice in equal proportion on the mixture surface. Stir after seasoning with salt and pepper.
3. Serve with or without tortilla chips.

NUTRITION INFORMATION

Calories 477

Fat 31g

Saturated Fat 4g

Cholesterol 99 mg

Sodium 305mg,

Carbohydrates 45g,

Fiber 15g,

Sugar 4g,

Protein 10g,

Calcium 10.1%

CHICKEN CAESAR SALAD ROLLED IN FLATBREAD

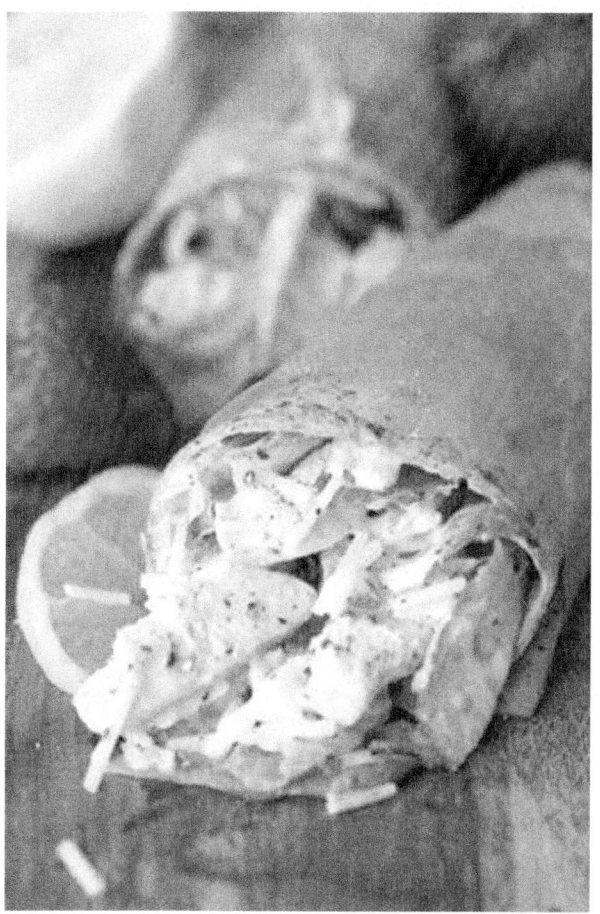

Total Prep Time: 25 Minutes

Yield: 5 serving

INGREDIENTS

- 8 chicken tenders
- 2 Tablespoons Olive Oil
- 8 cups romaine lettuce
- 1 ½ Cups of croutons
- ¾ Cup parmesan cheese grated

Flatbread Seasoning

- ¼ Cup Olive Oil
- 2 Cloves garlic minced
- 2 Tablespoons parsley
- ½ Cup parmesan cheese grated
- 4 Flatbreads

Dressing

- 1 Cup mayonnaise
- 2 garlic cloves minced
- 1 Tablespoon anchovy paste
- ¼ Cup parmesan cheese grated
- 2 teaspoons Worcestershire sauce
- 2 teaspoons Dijon mustard
- 3 Tablespoons lemon juice

INSTRUCTIONS

1. Mix all the dressing ingredients and set it aside.
2. Mix the chicken tenders with splashes of olive oil in a suitable bowl. Season as you like and grill it for 4-5 minutes on both sides until it is cooked thoroughly.
3. Whisk the olive oil with the garlic and parsley to create a paste. Gently using a brush or your fingers apply it on each side of the flatbread and grill it for a few minutes until it is lightly grilled. You can sprinkle some parmesan cheese on top and cook it until it melts.
4. Cut the lettuce into medium sized pieces. Next, Add the chicken, the parmesan cheese and the croutons then sprinkle your prepped dressing on top.
5. Finally, Cut your grilled flatbread into equal 6 pieces and serve it gracefully with the prepared salad.

NUTRITION INFORMATION:

Calories 1019

Fat 76g

Saturated Fat 16g

Cholesterol 116mg

Sodium 1586mg

Carbohydrates 38g

Fiber 3g

Sugar: 4g

Protein: 43g

Calcium: 54.3%

RICE SOUP

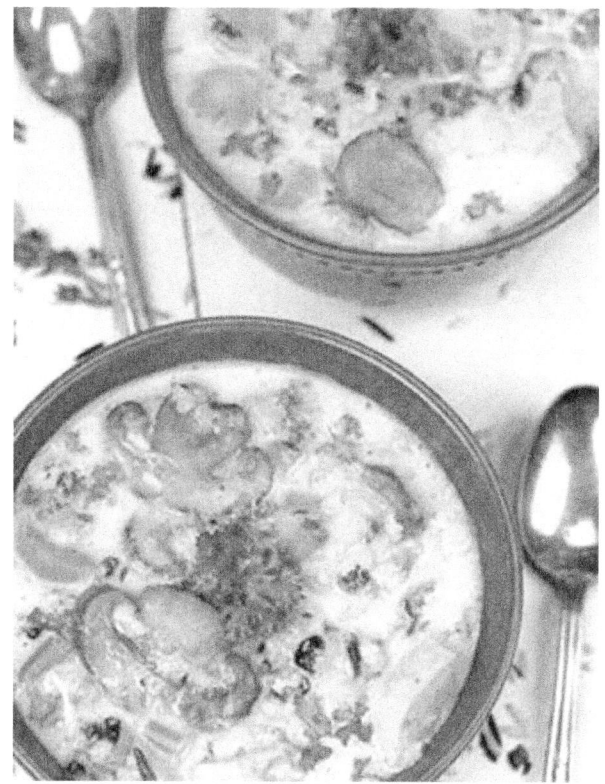

Total Prep Time: 1 Hour and 20 Minutes

Yields: 12 Serving

INGREDIENTS

- 2 Tablespoons Vegetable Oil

- 12 Ounces Cremini Mushrooms Trimmed and Sliced
- 2 Tablespoons Butter
- 1 Large Onion Chopped
- 4-6 Cloves Garlic Minced
- 4 Carrots Peeled and Diced
- 4 Celery Stalks Diced
- ¼ Cup All-Purpose Flour
- 64 Ounces Low Sodium Chicken Broth
- 1 Teaspoon Dried Thyme
- 1 ½ Tablespoons "Better Than Bouillon"-Chicken Flavor
- 1 ½ Cups Wild Rice Blend
- 1 ½ Cups Frozen Corn Thawed and Well Drained
- 4 Cups Chicken or Turkey Cooked and Cubed
- 1 Cup Heavy Cream
- 2 Tablespoons Fresh Parsley Chopped

INSTRUCTIONS

1. Using a Dutch oven, heat the olive oil over medium heat. Next, add mushrooms cutlets and stir until they begin to darken for around 5-8 minutes then put aside.
2. Add butter, then add the garlic, onion, carrots, and celery with butter until they start to soften. Combine the cooked

mushrooms to the vegetable mix and add flour then let it cook 1 minute while continuing to stir.

3. To the mixture, add the following: The Better than Bouillon, thyme, the Wild rice blend, and broth and season with one and half a teaspoon salt and one teaspoon pepper then let it boil.

4. When it boils, lower the heat from medium to low and it simmer while keeping it partially covered, then let it cook till the rice is becomes cooked and tender which takes about half an hour. You can then pour in the remaining ingredients and let it all simmer for the flavors to be absorbed for about 10 to 15 minutes.

NUTRITION INFORMATION

Calories: 181

Fat: 12g

Saturated Fat: 7g

Cholesterol: 32mg

Sodium: 97mg

Potassium: 453mg

Carbohydrates: 14g

Fiber: 1g

Sugar: 2g

Protein: 5g

Calcium: 4.2%

LEMON CHICKEN SOUP

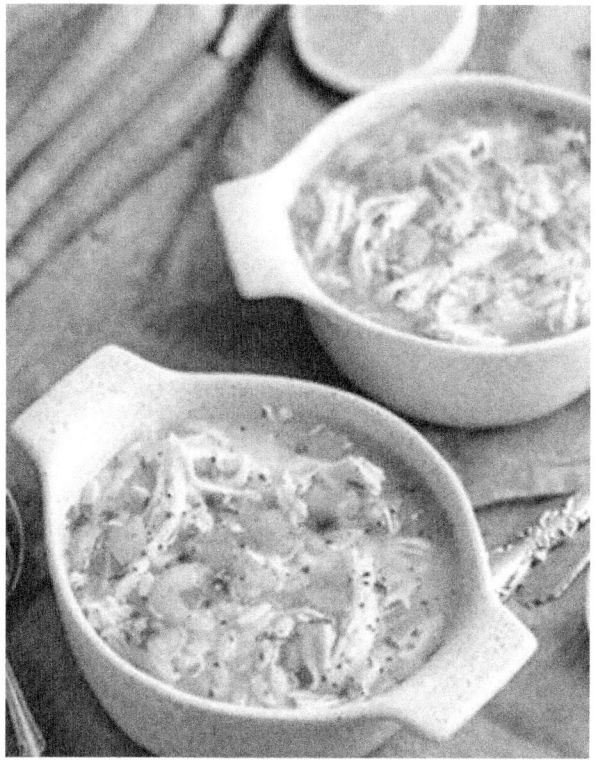

Total Prep Time: 25 minutes

Yield: 4 servings

INGREDIENTS

- 1 Tablespoon of virgin olive oil

- 2 Tablespoons of unsalted butter (separate)
- 2 chicken breasts trimmed of fat (boneless)
- ½ Teaspoon kosher salt
- ¼ Teaspoon black pepper
- 1 medium yellow onion diced
- 2 medium carrots peeled and diced
- 1 large celery stalk diced
- 4 cloves garlic minced
- ½ Teaspoon dried thyme
- 4 cups chicken broth reduced sodium
- 1 ½ Cups water
- 1 cup dried uncooked orzo pasta
- 1 bay leaf
- 1 sprig fresh rosemary
- 1 sprig fresh oregano
- Juice of 1 lemon
- 2 teaspoons minced fresh parsley

INSTRUCTIONS

1. You can cook in a large Dutch oven or a stockpot. Over medium heat, heat the olive oil and one tablespoon of butter

2. Flavor the chicken with salt and pepper to taste on each side of chicken breast then place it in the Dutch oven and let it cook for 3-4 minutes each side and until you see its color change to golden brown. Remove the chicken and put it aside.

3. You can add rest of the butter to the Dutch oven and combine it with carrots, celery, garlic, and onion, then cook it all together until they soften and make sure you frequently stir then finally add the dried thyme.

4. Add the chicken broth and the adequate water amount and let it boil, when the chicken softens, you can shred the chicken to smaller pieces with a fork. Add the remaining ingredients such as rosemary and oregano and let it all simmer to absorb the flavor, however, don't forget to filter out the leaves of rosemary and oregano.

5. You can add lemon juice and fresh parsley.

NUTRITION INFORMATION

Calories: 217

Fat: 7g

Saturated Fat: 3g

Cholesterol: 34mg

Sodium: 831mg

Carbohydrates: 24g

Fiber: 1g

Sugar: 2g

Protein: 12g

Calcium: 3.8%

SUMMER BERRIES MEDLEY

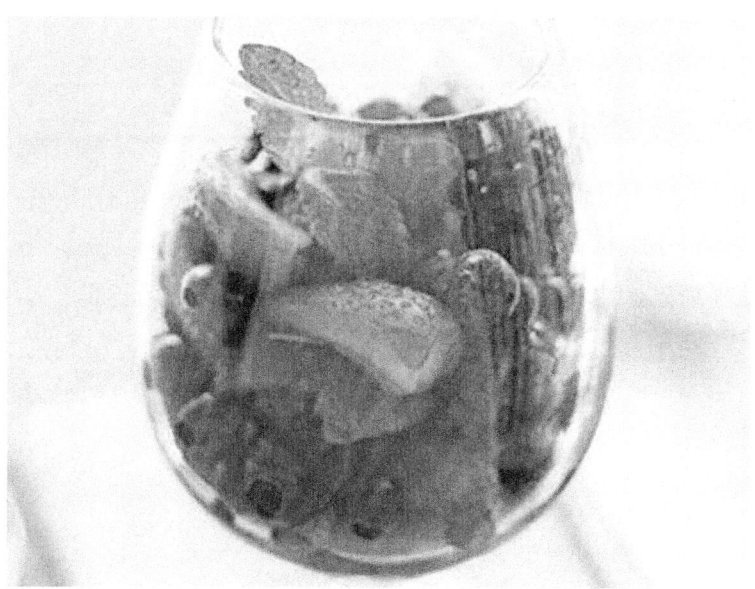

Total Prep Time: 10 Minutes

Yields: 6 Serving

INGREDIENTS

- 2 tablespoons fresh lemon juice

- 1 tablespoon grated lemon rind

- 1/2 cup torn mint leaves

- 1 cup fresh raspberries

- 2 cups hulled fresh strawberries

- 2 cups fresh blackberries

- 1/4 cup sugar

- quartered 2 cups fresh blueberries

INSTRUCTIONS

In a glass cup or bowl, combine all the ingredients together, add your mint then stir well.

NUTRITIONAL INFORMATION

Calories 136

Fat 0.8g

Sat fat 0.0g

Cholesterol 0.0mg

Sodium 2 mg

Carbohydrate 31.3g

Fiber 7.4g

Sugar 4 g

Protein 1.9g

Calcium 38mg

GREEK SALMON BOWL

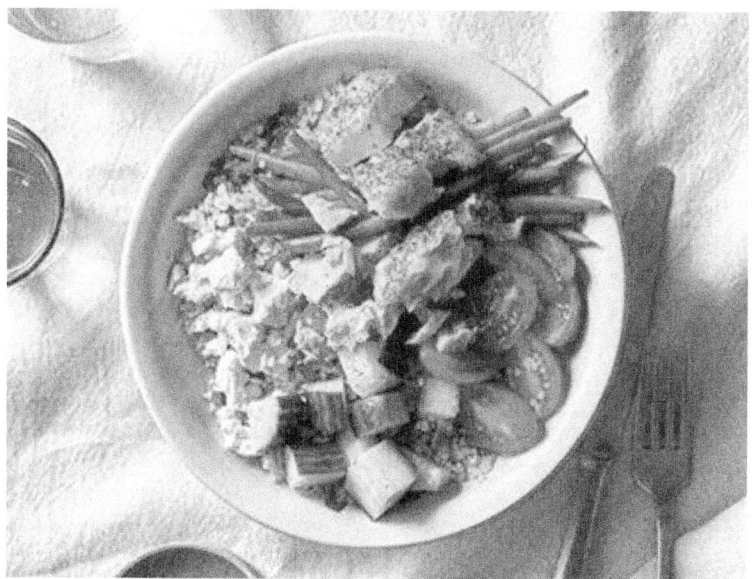

Total Prep Time: 20 Minutes

Yields: 4 servings

INGREDIENTS

- 1/2 cup chopped fresh flat-leaf parsley
- 3 cups of baby spinach leaves, finely chopped
- 1 teaspoon kosher salt
- 5 tablespoons canola oil, divided

- 4 (5-oz.) skin-on salmon fillets
- 1/2 teaspoon dried dill
- 1/2 teaspoon dried oregano divided
- 1 (8-oz.) pkg. haricots verts
- 1 1/2 cups cooked quinoa
- 1/4 cup fresh lemon juice
- 1 teaspoon honey
- 2 cups halved grape tomatoes
- 2 cups chopped English cucumber
- 1/4 cup crumbled feta cheese

INSTRUCTIONS

1. Add the dill, oregano, and 1/4 teaspoon of salt to the salmon.

2. In a large non-stick cooking utensil, heat 1 tablespoon oil over medium heat then place the salmon in the skillet and grill for 2 to 3 minutes each side then keep it aside.

3. Follow the package instructions on the haricots verts package to cook then place in a bowl full of ice cold water to drop their temperature one minute then dry it.

4. To create a spinach mixture, combine the parsley, spinach and quinoa.

5. Prepare the dressing by mixing the lemon with honey and the remaining oil. Take a quarter of the dressing and add it to the spinach mixture.

6. Serve in each bowl 3/4 cup of the spinach mixture then distribute the tomatoes, haricot verts, cucumbers and the remaining dressing equally in each bowl. Add one salmon fillet to each bowl which you can top with one tablespoon of feta cheese.

NUTRITIONAL INFORMATION

Calories 527

Fat 29g

Sat fat 5g

Cholesterol 0 mg

Sodium 683mg

Protein 39g

Carbohydrate 29g

Fiber 7g

Sugars 8g

Calcium 16%

BARELY AND BERRY GRANOLA (TOASTED)

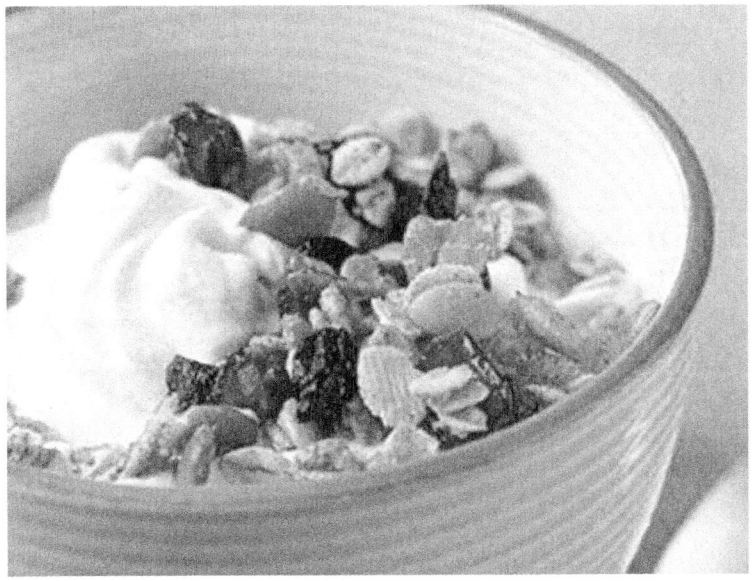

Total Prep Time: 35 Minutes

Yields: 4 serving

INGREDIENTS

- 1/4 cup unsalted pumpkinseed kernels
- 1/3 cup dried blueberries
- 1/3 cup maple syrup

- 2 tablespoons canola oil
- 1 teaspoon ground cinnamon
- 1/8 teaspoon ground cardamom
- 1 1/2 teaspoons vanilla extract
- 1/4 teaspoon salt
- 2 tablespoons brown sugar
- 1/3 cup sweetened dried cranberries
- 2 cups rolled barley flakes
- 1/4 cup toasted wheat germ
- 1/4 cup unsalted sunflower seed kernels

INSTRUCTIONS

1. While you prep your ingredients preheat the oven to 325 F.
2. In a baking sheet, bake the kernel sunflower seeds and the pumpkin seed kernels and bake for 5 minutes to toast then let them cool afterwards.
3. Mix the syrup with the vanilla extract, canola oil, brown sugar, cinnamon, a pinch of salt and the ground cardamom and stir.
4. Add the barley, and wheat germ as well as the toasted kernels to the syrup mixture and stir.

5. On a baking sheet, spread the mixture as a single layer and let it bake for 25 minutes while making sure to stir every 10 minutes.

6. Once it becomes golden brown, take it out of the oven and let it cool. Then mix in your berries and store in a sealed container for a healthy breakfast.

NUTRITIONAL INFORMATION

Calories 181

Fat 6.5g

Sat fat 0.7g

Cholesterol 1mg

Protein 4.5g

Carbohydrate 27.4g

Fiber 3.7g

Sugar 3 g

Sodium 59mg

Calcium 13mg

EASY OAT MEAL BREAKFAST

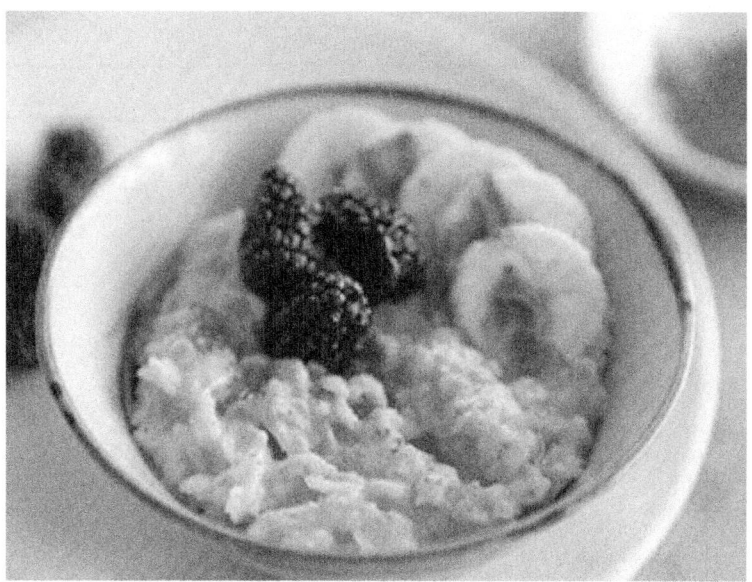

Total Prep Time: 7 Minutes

Yields: 2 servings

INGREDIENTS

- 1 cup of oats
- 1 cup milk
- 1 teaspoon honey
- 1 cup of water

- 1/2 teaspoon ground cinnamon
- 1/8 teaspoon kosher salt
- Toppings, as desired, could be nuts, berries, etc or fresh fruit)

INSTRUCTIONS

1. In a suitable saucepan, add the oats and mix with the milk, salt, water, and cinnamon. Let it boil, then decrease the heat.
2. Allow it to simmer for three to five minutes until it becomes thick, keep stirring every once in a while, then remove it off the heat and allow it to cool slowly.
3. Proportion your mixture equally among the bowls and add some honey to each serving. You can top off your dish with berries or any desired toppings.

NUTRITIONAL INFORMATION

Calories 220

Fat 5g

Sat fat 2g

Cholesterol 1 mg

Sodium 180mg

Protein 12g

Carbohydrates 36g

Fiber 4g

Sugars 10g

Calcium 15%

AVOCADO AND STRAWBERRY SALAD WITH TORTILLA CHIPS

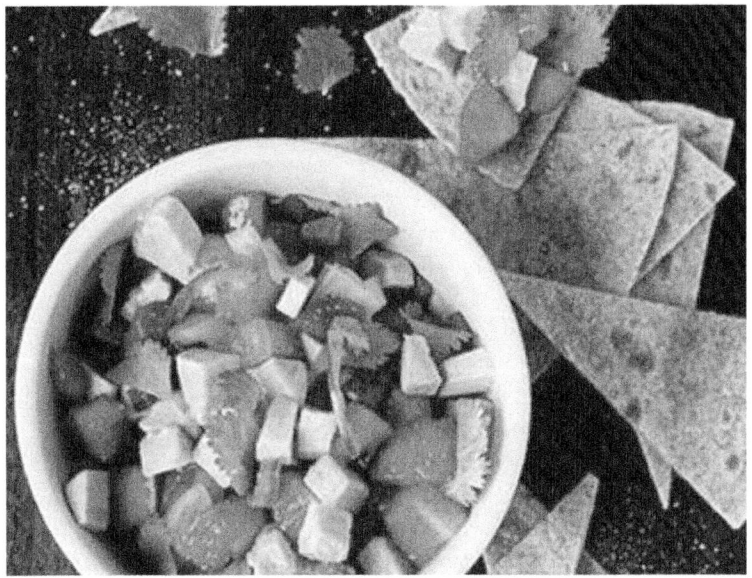

Total Prep Time: 7 Minutes

Yields: 2 servings

INGREDIENTS

- 2 teaspoons canola oil
- 6 (6-inch) whole-wheat flour tortillas
- 1/2 teaspoon ground cinnamon

- 2 teaspoons sugar
- 1 cup finely chopped strawberries
- 1 1/2 cups of neatly chopped and peeled ripe avocado (2 Avocados)
- 2 tablespoons minced fresh cilantro
- 3/8 teaspoon salt
- 1 teaspoon minced seeded jalapeño pepper
- 2 teaspoons fresh lime juice

INSTRUCTIONS

1. Start by preheating the oven to 350°.
2. Prime your tortilla by gently brushing the oil equally on each side of the tortilla chip.
3. Mix the sugar with the cinnamon to make a nice garnish and sprinkle it equally on the tortilla sides; the oil will help the mix to stick to the tortilla.
4. Divide using a knife, each tortilla into twelve wedge-shaped pieces and put them in one layer over two baking sheets then place it in the preheated oven and bake for 10 minutes until they start to feel crispy.
5. Mix the avocado with the remaining ingredients to create the salad and stir adequately to mingle the ingredients then serve gracefully with the baked chips.

NUTRITIONAL INFORMATION

Calories 138

Fat 6.7g

Sat Fat 1g

Cholesterol 0.0 mg

Protein 2.8g

Carbohydrate 17.3g

Sugars 4 g

Fiber 3.6g

Sodium 246mg

Calcium 7mg

BLACKBERRY SMOOTHIE

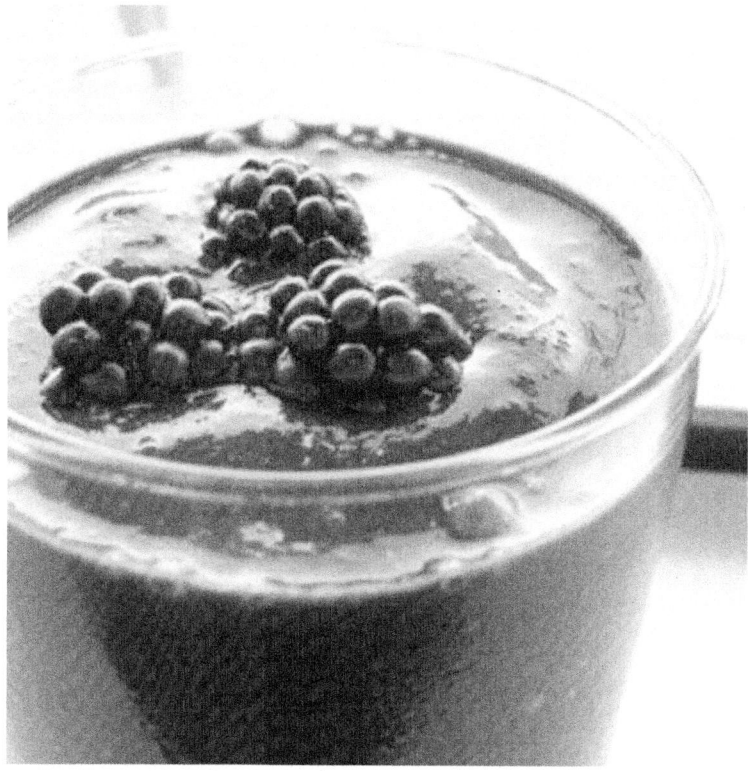

Total Prep Time: 7 Minutes

Yield: 2 servings

INGREDIENTS

- 2 cups fresh or frozen blackberries

- 1 cup plain fat-free yoghurt
- 1 large ripe banana
- 1 cup apple juice
- 1/4 cup honey

INSTRUCTIONS

1. Mix all the ingredients in a blender.
2. Let it all blend until you got a smooth texture.
3. Using a sieve, run your smoothie to get rid of all the seeds or hard lumps.
4. Serve with ice cubes if desired.

NUTRITIONAL INFORMATION

Calories 264

Calories from fat 3%

Fat 0.7g

Sat fat 0.2g

Protein 5.6g

Carbohydrate 63.2g

Fiber 8.8g

Cholesterol 2mg

Sodium 62mg

Calcium 192mg

BEST SUPER FOODS FOR IMMUNITY

Having a strong immune system also means that you are very healthy. Whether you're trying to prevent the flu that has affected everyone around you or avoid catching a cold, you will obviously need a strong and healthy immune system. Sure, washing your hands, getting a flu shot or staying away from coughing people will protect you. But somehow the virus or bacteria will find its way to your body.

That's where your immune system steps in. That said, you need to strengthen your immune system and there's no better way than eating the right foods. In this article, I will show you the best foods that will improve your immunity.

How We Get Sick and How We Heal?

The health of our body is very important, that is why we have many defense systems in place. The first defense system is your intact skin, that seals off the inner environment of your body from any invading, harmful microorganisms. However, there are many other routes that bacteria and other diseases causing organisms can get into your body, for example, via inhalation from the air, via poor hand hygiene or from eating contaminated food.

In that case, you need an inner defense system to protect your body from those invading pathogens as they will multiply if nothing stops them. This is how we get sick, when harmful organisms get inside our body, start to multiply and release their harmful toxic substances inside our bodies.

This is the role of your inner immunity; to protect you from these organisms. It does this by first detecting an invasion, then releasing inflammatory substances which alerts other immunity cells known as the white blood cells to come and attack the pathogen.

The white blood cells trap the pathogens to contain the infection and limit its spread. They also kill off the pathogens by releasing antioxidant substances.

There are a number of foods you can eat that can provide your body with natural compounds that will help boost your immunity, support your white blood cell function and production. If you are having repeated infections, after you visit your doctor, it is time to start eating immunity boosting food. Let us look at some examples of immunity boosting super foods:

1. Poultry

If you had parents like mine, I'm sure you remember chicken soup. The minute I had a cold, my parents always cooked chicken soup to help soothe the symptoms. Chicken soup also helps to protect you from getting sick in the first place.

Chicken and turkey, for example, have a high concentration of Vitamin B-6 which is vital for the formation of red blood cells. On top of that, poultry has high concentrations of gelatin and other nutrients in their bones which are helpful in healing the gut and immunity.

The nutrients in chicken soup are also the ultimate solution to receive a healthy dose of anti-inflammatory substance that helps your body to fight infections.

2. Citrus fruits

Most citrus fruits for instance lemons have a high concentration of Vitamin C. Vitamin C is a key player in your immunity. Some infections cannot be treated by antibiotics and you would need your body's immunity to come into play. Here comes the critical role of Vitamin C. It increases the production of white blood cells that will fight off the cold. White blood cells are the key immunity cells that kill of pathogens and attack them. More importantly, your body is not able to store Vitamin C. Therefore, you need to eat food rich in vitamin C on a daily basis.

Example of citrus fruits are any fruit that kind of tastes sour, like lemon, oranges, tangerines, etc.

3. Broccoli

If you have been suffering from repeated infections, it is a sign that your immunity is low, so it is time to bring some powerful immunity boosters to the table, for example, broccoli.

Broccoli is packed with vitamins A, E and C together with other antioxidants. This vegetable will give your immune system a serious boost due to the combined effect of these three nutrients in raising your body's natural immunity and fighting off inflammation via the powerful anti-oxidant effect. The vitamins are powerful antioxidants that will help your body to fight off infection.

4. Garlic

This is one of the most common home-made remedies to raise immunity and fight repeated infections. It helps fight off colds and other diseases. That's because garlic contains allicin which reduces the effects of cold. Allicin is highly unstable so it converts into a compound that is thought to give garlic its medicinal properties. It contains natural bactericidal properties via its sulphur containing products. These natural compounds help to flush your body and raise your immunity.

5. Green tea

Most people enjoy green tea as an alternative to taking coffee or black tea. That's because it contains trace amounts of caffeine compared to the rest. On top of that, green tea also contains flavonoid and powerful antioxidants which fight off the inflammation resulting from infections, therefore, helping your symptoms to disappear quickly. It contains the powerful antioxidant epigallocatechin gallate, or EGCG which is a compound that strengthens your immunity and reduces the effects of diseases such as colds by curbing the inflammatory cascade and damaging effects of infections. It also aids in the production of components that help the WBC fight infections better.

6. Ginger

Enjoyed in most desserts, ginger packs a lot of nutrients that also boost your immunity. That's because ginger has antioxidant properties that will help you fight off free radicals. More to that, ginger also has anti-inflammatory properties that will help you heal faster and speed up the process. If you have a sore throat, ginger is your go-to drink.

On top of that, ginger also helps counteract that nausea feeling that you've been struggling with. It is able to soothe the stomach and aid in the digestion process all which will keep your body in a good condition and help your body focus on fighting any incoming infections.

7. Oranges

If you suffer from repeated infections, you can easily snack on oranges or have an orange drink for boosted immunity. Oranges are an excellent source of vitamin C. When it comes to suffering from cold, vitamin C is the best solution. It will help you deal with your illness easily. Research has also shown that vitamin C reduces the symptoms of the disease as well as the duration you will suffer from it. That is because it supports the production of white blood cells which ward off infections.

8. Turmeric

Turmeric tea is the best way to enjoy a cup of tea while boosting your immune system. Known for its anti-inflammatory properties, turmeric tea will ensure that you have a stable and strong immune system. It is one of the most ancient remedies to help strengthen the immune system naturally and fend against any bacteria via its bactericidal effects.

It can also act as an anti-microbial agent in your body. One of the most important compounds is the curcumin which is not easily absorbed by the body. You need to help your body by eating turmeric. Curcumin is able to kill bacteria.

9. Spinach

This is another food that will also boost your immune system. Spinach contains flavonoids, Vitamin C and E, and carotenoids which help support your immunity. Carotenoids are a powerful antioxidant that is easily converted by the body to Vitamin A which is vital for growth and immune functions. The antioxidant function is needed by your white blood cells to kill the invading pathogens.

Vitamin C and E are also strong anti-oxidants that help the body to fight off any infection.

10. Almond

And finally, almonds are an excellent source of vitamin E. on top of that; they also contain fibre, magnesium, and manganese. Vitamin E is a strong antioxidant that helps preserve the muscles and the red blood cells. It also boosts the response of vaccines when it comes to protecting your body against infection.

Magnesium also boosts your immunity by strengthening your bones and muscles while supporting other body functions.

Top Super food Recipes for Immunity

ORANGE TEA

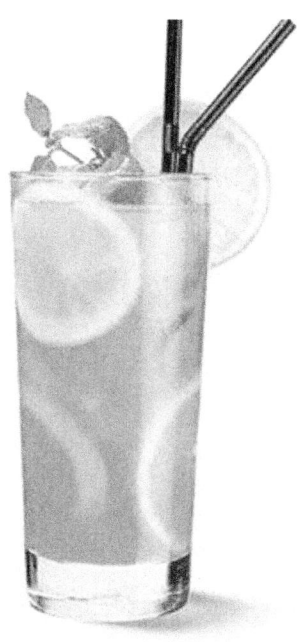

Total Prep Time: 5 Minutes

Yield: 1 Serving

INGREDIENTS

- ½ cup of orange juice
- 1 cup of cold water
- 3 black tea bags
- ¼ cup sugar
- 4 tablespoon thinly sliced orange
- 3-4 mints for garnishing
- 1 cup boiling water
- Orange wedge 3-4

INSTRUCTIONS

1. Pour the tea bags and sliced orange into boiling water for 3 to 5 minutes.
2. Strain the tea and pour into a large pitcher.
3. Add orange juice and sugar stir the sugar until it gets dissolved.
4. Add cold water.
5. Refrigerate the tea and serve it with orange wedges and garnish it with mint leaves.

NUTRITIONAL INFORMATION

35 calories

0 g fat

0 g sat

3 g fiber

9 g carbohydrates

0 g protein

0mg cholesterol

6 g added sugars

6 mg calcium

5 mg sodium

ALMOND GREEN BEANS

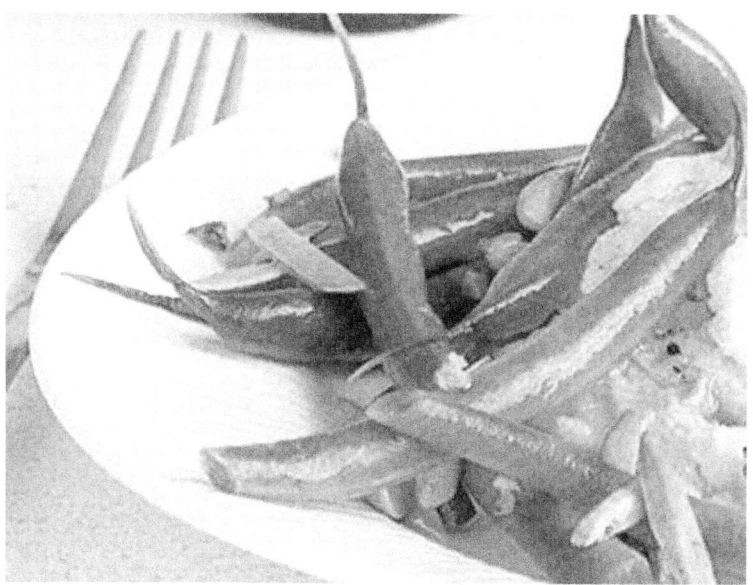

Total Prep Time: 25 Minutes

Yield: 4 Servings

INGREDIENTS

- 1 tablespoon butter
- 1/4 cup slivered almonds
- 2 teaspoons minced fresh garlic
- 12 ounces trimmed green beans

- 3 tablespoons water
- 1/4 teaspoon salt
- 1/4 teaspoon freshly ground black pepper

INSTRUCTIONS

1. Melt the butter in a skillet over average heat.
2. Add the almonds and cook for 2 to 3 minutes or until they turn into lightly browned color. Keep stirring frequently.
3. Remove the fried almond from the pan. Add some garlic to the pot and stir, let it cook for 30 seconds.
4. Add the green beans, salt to taste, the water, and pepper.
5. Place the lid on the pan and cook for 4 minutes or until beans are cooked, and the liquid evaporates. Sprinkle with almonds.

NUTRITIONAL INFORMATION

Calories 93

Fat 6.4g

Sat fat 2.1g

Cholesterol 0.2 g

Sodium 178mg

Carbohydrates 5 grams

Sugar 1 g

Fiber 4

Calcium 6%

BROCCOLI SOUP

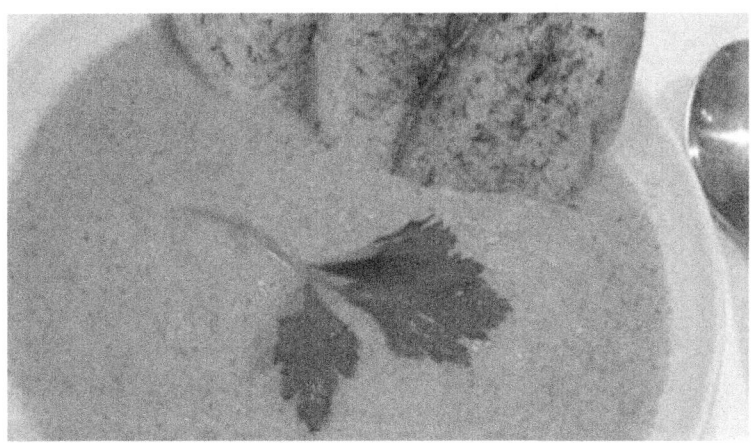

Total Prep Time: 25 Minutes

Yield: 5 Servings

INGREDIENTS

- 1 tablespoon olive oil
- 1 large onion, chopped
- 1 potato, peeled and chopped
- 3 cloves garlic, peeled and chopped
- 20 ounces of broccoli
- 4 cups chicken broth

- 1/4 teaspoon ground nutmeg
- Salt and pepper to taste

INSTRUCTIONS

1. Heat and oil a suitable pan.
2. Fry the onion and garlic until it becomes soft and golden.
3. Mix in the broccoli and potato and pour in the chicken broth.
4. Let it boil then drop the heat and allow it to simmer for 15 minutes till you feel the vegetables turn soft.
5. Using a blender or a hand mixture, puree the mixture until smooth.
6. Return the smooth pour into the saucepan to reheat — season with nutmeg, salt, and pepper.

NUTRITIONAL INFORMATION

Calories 64

Fat 2g

Carbohydrates 11g

Fiber 8 G

Sugars 3 G

Protein 2.8

Cholesterol 0 Mg

Sodium 20 Mg

Calcium 6%

ROASTED BROCCOLI WITH GARLIC

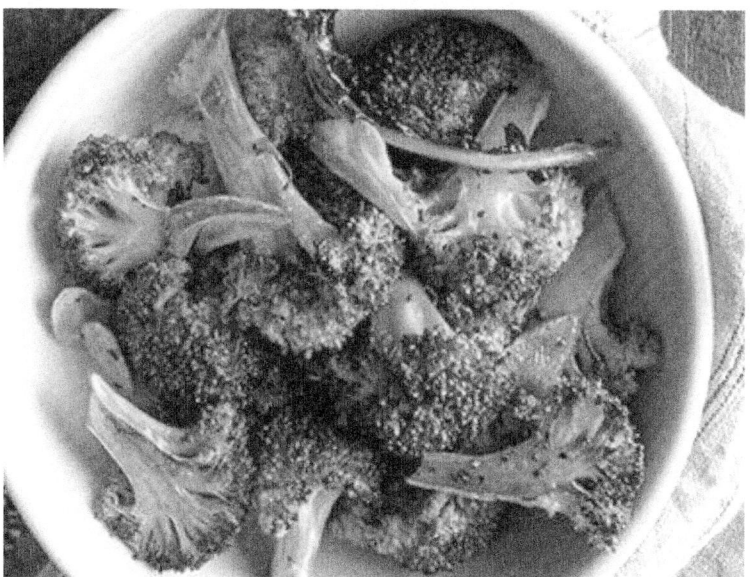

Total Prep Time: 35 Minutes

Yield: 6 Servings

INGREDIENTS

- 4-5 pounds broccoli
- 4 garlic cloves peeled and thinly sliced
- 1½ teaspoons kosher salt
- 5 tablespoons of olive oil

- ½ teaspoon freshly ground black pepper
- 2 teaspoons grated lemon zest
- 2 tablespoons freshly squeezed lemon juice
- ⅓ cup freshly grated Parmesan cheese

INSTRUCTIONS

1. Preheat the oven to 425 degrees F.
2. Cut the broccoli into florets and remove the thick stalks but you can leave an inch or two of stalk still attached to the florets.
3. Put the cut broccoli florets on a baking sheet in one layer.
4. Add the garlic to the broccoli and drizzle about 5 tablespoons olive oil. Add the salt and pepper to taste.
5. Let it bake for 25 minutes until some of the florets have browned.
6. Remove the broccoli from the oven and immediately toss with 1 1/2 tablespoons olive oil, the lemon zest, lemon juice, and Parmesan. Serve hot.

NUTRITIONAL INFORMATION

Calories 129

Total Fat 2g

Saturated Fat 1g

Cholesterol 3mg

Sodium 770mg

Carbohydrates 21g

Fiber 8g

Sugars 5g

Protein 10g

Calcium 21.2%

Iron 12.7%

GINGER TUMERIC TEA

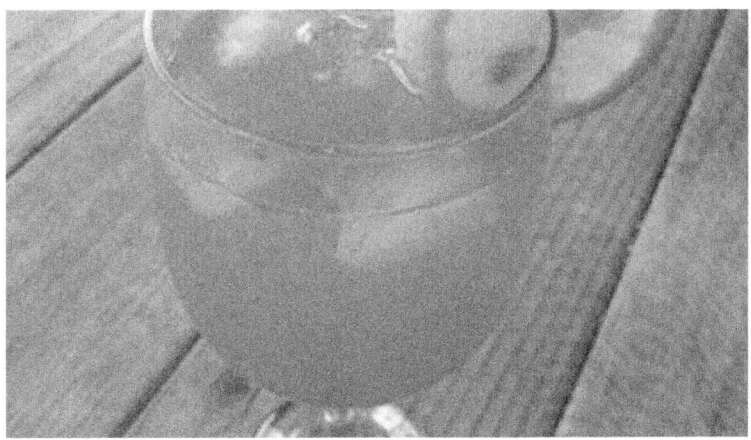

Total Prep Time: 20 Minutes

Yield: 1 Serving

INGREDIENTS

- 2 cups of water
- 1/2 teaspoon ground turmeric
- 1/2 teaspoon chopped fresh ginger
- 1/2 teaspoon ground cinnamon (optional)
- 1 tablespoon honey
- 1 lemon wedge

INSTRUCTIONS

1. Boil Water.
2. Add the turmeric, ginger, and cinnamon.
3. Lower heat and leave it to simmer for ten minutes.
4. Strain tea into a large glass; add the honey and a lemon wedge.

NUTRITIONAL INFORMATION

Calories 37

Fat 0.1 g

Saturated fats 0

Carbohydrates 10.3 g

Protein 0.2 g

Cholesterol 0

Sodium 8 mg

SUNSHINE ORANGE SMOOTHIE

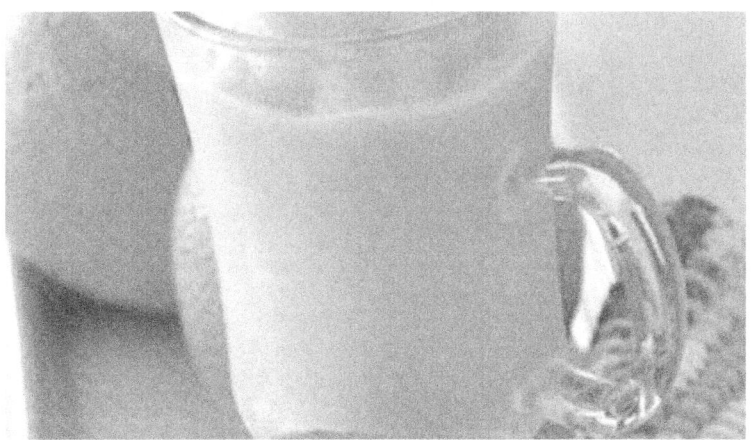

Total Prep Time: 3 Minutes

Yield: 1 Serving

INGREDIENTS

- 1 mango - peeled, seedless, and cut into chunks
- 1 banana, peeled and chopped
- 1 cup orange juice
- 1 cup vanilla nonfat yoghurt

INSTRUCTIONS

1. Place mango, orange juice, banana, and yoghurt in a blender.
2. Pulse until smooth.
3. Serve in clear glasses, and drink with a bendy straw!

NUTRITIONAL INFORMATION

151 calories

0.5 g fat

34.6 g carbohydrates

4.2 g protein

< 1 mg cholesterol

44 mg sodium

BLT Pasta Salad

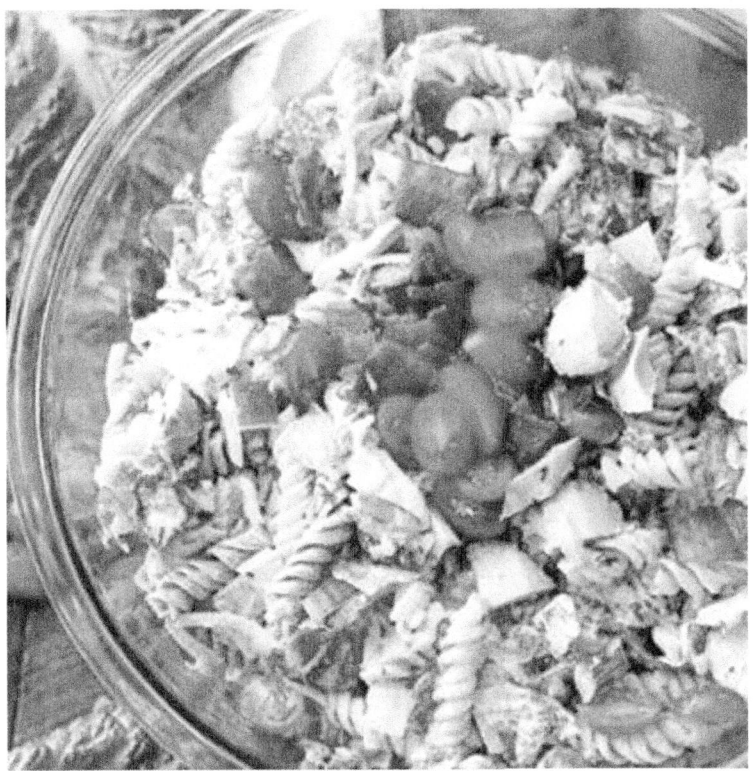

Total Prep Time: 25 Minutes

Yield: 5 servings

INGREDIENTS

- 10 slices of bacon cooked and diced, greased on both sides
- 12 oz of pasta cooked and cooled
- ½ Cup mayonnaise
- ¾ Cup ranch dressing homemade ranch is best
- 1 ½ Cup diced tomatoes
- ½ Avocado diced
- 1 cup cheddar cheese shredded
- 1/3 Cup red onion diced
- 1 cup romaine lettuce
- Fresh parsley for garnish optional

INSTRUCTIONS

1. Mix together the mayonnaise, the ranch dressing and 1 tablespoon bacon grease (optional).
2. In a suitable bowl assemble the pasta, tomatoes, avocado, cheese, red onion, lettuce and bacon.
3. Drizzle the prepped dressing over the mixture and toss around to combine.
4. Garnish with parsley and serve.

NUTRITIONAL INFORMATION

Calories 502

Fat 32g

 Saturated Fat 9g

Cholesterol 42mg

Sodium 628mg

Carbohydrates 38g

Fiber 3g

Sugar 3g

Protein 13g

Calcium 13.8%

LEMON CHICKEN

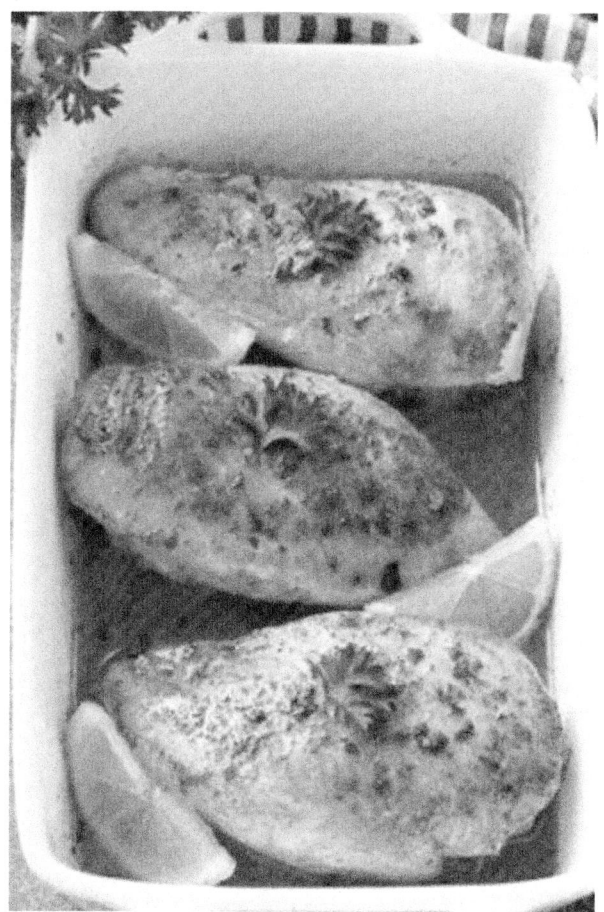

Total Prep Time: 35 Minutes

Yield: 4 Servings

INGREDIENTS

- 4 skinless and boneless chicken breasts (about 1 1/2 lb.)
- 1/2 teaspoon pepper
- 1 teaspoon salt
- 1/3 cup all-purpose flour
- 8 lemon slices
- 4 tablespoons butter, divided
- 2 tablespoons olive oil, divided
- 1/4 cup chicken broth
- 1/4 cup lemon juice
- 1/4 cup chopped parsley
- Garnish: lemon slices

INSTRUCTIONS

1. Using a knife cut each of your chicken breasts in half and season with salt and pepper then gently sprinkle some flour on it and shake off the excess flour.

2. Over a hot oiled skillet, cook your chicken breasts for a couple of minutes until done. Repeat till all breasts are cooked and set aside.

3. In the same skillet, pour in the broth and lemon juice and stir. Cook for 1-2 minutes. Add some of the slices of lemon.

4. To the above mix, add the remaining butter and the parsley and stir till the butter melts.

5. Pour this sauce with the chicken and serve hot.

NUTRITIONAL INFORMATION

Calories 226

Total Fat 12 g

Saturated fat 1.9 g

Cholesterol 32 mg

Sodium 243 mg

Carbohydrate 19 g

fiber 1.1 g

Sugar 9 g

Protein 11 g

Calcium 12 %

ALMOND SPINACH SALAD

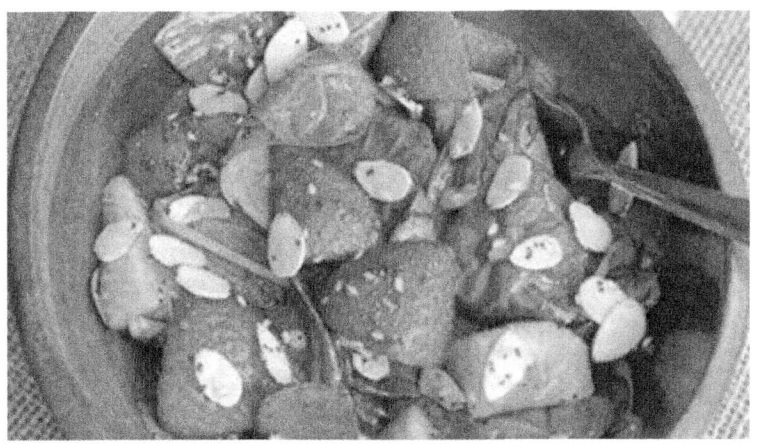

Total Prep Time: 20 Minutes

Yield: 4 Servings

INGREDIENTS

- 2 tablespoons sesame seeds
- 1 tablespoon poppy seeds
- 1/2 cup olive oil
- 1/2 cup white sugar
- 1/4 teaspoon Worcestershire sauce
- 1/4 cup distilled white vinegar
- 1/4 teaspoon paprika

- 1 tablespoon minced onion
- 1-quart strawberries - cleaned, hulled and sliced
- 10 ounces of fresh spinach - rinsed well, dried and torn into bite-size pieces
- 1/4 cup almonds, blanched and slivered

INSTRUCTIONS

1. In a suitable bowl, mix well together with the sesame and poppy seeds, along with the onion, and pour in the olive oil, vinegar and sprinkle paprika and sugar and add some Worcestershire sauce.
2. Lid the mixture and allow it to chill for one hour.
3. In another bowl, add the spinach with the strawberries and the almonds.
4. Add the prepared dressing over your salad and mix well.
5. Refrigerate to chill for 10 to 15 minutes before you serve.

NUTRITIONAL INFORMATION

491 calories

35.2 g fat

42.9 g carbohydrates

6 g protein

0 mg cholesterol

63 mg sodium

Calcium 10.3%

MIDDLE EASTERN CARROT SALAD

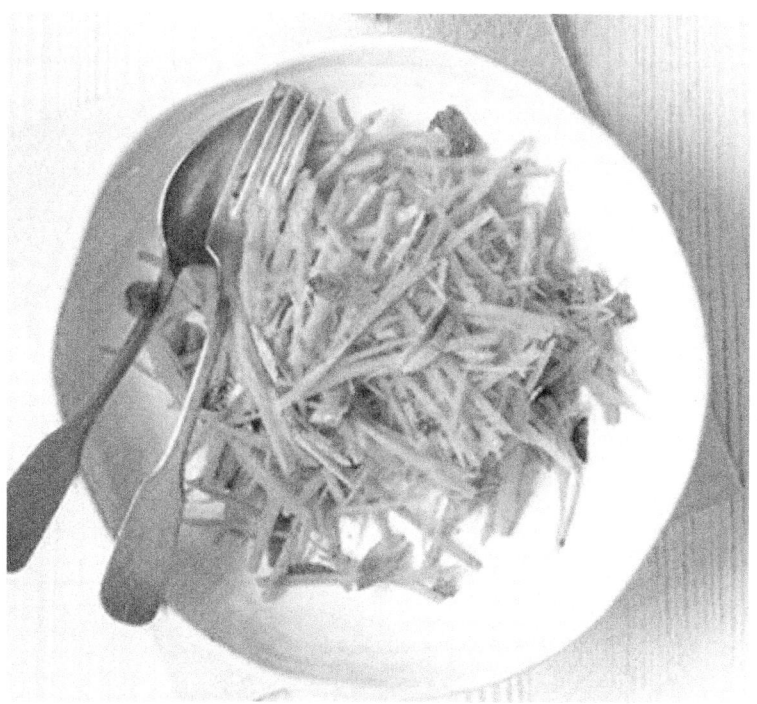

Total Prep Time: 10 Minutes

Yield: 4 Servings

INGREDIENTS

- ½ tsp orange blossom water
- ½ tsp ground cumin

- 1 tbsp extra virgin olive oil
- ½ lemon juice
- 500g carrot (shredded or grated large handful small mint)

INSTRUCTIONS

1. Pour in the orange blossom water and add to it the cumin, oil, lemon juice and some seasoning into a jar. Screw the lid tightly and shake well to mix.
2. Take the grated carrots and add it along with mint into a bowl.
3. Pour over the dressing from the jar and season and toss around to combine everything together.

NUTRITIONAL INFORMATION

Calories: 217

Fat: 7g

Saturated Fat: 3g

Cholesterol: 34mg

Sodium: 831mg

Carbohydrates: 24g

Fiber: 1g

Sugar: 2g

Protein: 12g

Calcium: 3.8%

Best Super Foods for Thyroid Health

The thyroid gland is a silent powerhouse that always goes unnoticed despite its importance. It is a butterfly-shaped gland found in your neck. It is a relatively small gland. However, that doesn't reduce its importance in our bodies. The thyroid controls your heartbeat, metabolism, temperature and so much more. It does this by producing a hormone called the thyroid hormone. This hormone is carried in our blood to lots of our body tissues and organs where it influences the function of that organ.

Most of all, in case anything goes wrong in this gland, you will definitely notice. When your thyroid gland fails to produce enough thyroid hormone, you most likely will be suffering from hypothyroidism. This is a medical condition that includes a long list of manifest symptoms. There is a wide range of symptoms that emerge if the thyroid fails, as it has a role with various body systems and the thyroid hormone control various bodily processes including sweating, alertness, body weight, heart rate and much more.

If your thyroid fails to activate these functions, you may experience some of the following symptoms:

- Puffy Face,

- Slow, slurred speech

- Confusion, depression and difficulty to concentrate

- Excessive sensitivity to cold

- Cramps and fatigue

- Changes in your body hair texture or amount than usual

- Weight gain

- Slow pulse and decreased heart rate

If you are feeling a combination of these symptoms, it is time to visit your doctor and further investigation. If you do indeed suffer from hypothyroidism, you need to start providing your thyroid with all it needs to support the production and release of the thyroid hormone. There is a number of ways you can support your thyroid's health, but the best one natural one is via eating food rich in iodine that can improve your thyroid health and support healthy hormone production levels.

What are the essential items needed for healthy thyroid hormone production?

Iodine is integral to the production of the thyroid hormone. Inadequate production of the thyroid hormone leads to medical conditions such as goitre and hypothyroidism. Goitre is the enlargement of the thyroid gland in an attempt to compensate for the low production level (the body's logic is if you have a bigger gland, you can produce more to compensate for the inadequacy of the hormone). However, the number one reason for the inadequate production is a deficiency of iodine which is integral to the production of the thyroid hormone.

Here are the best super foods that can help you with that:

1. Milk

A high percentage of iodine in our diets come from milk products. If you drink one cup of milk every single day, you will have covered at least one-third of your daily iodine needs, see, it is that simple!

Milk can help you prevent against hypothyroidism, however, if you are on medication for thyroid, the calcium in the milk can interfere with your medicine. Therefore, you need to be cautious about how much milk you consume. Moreover, try not to have milk close to your medication time.

If you suffer from GIT problems, the casein in mil can be hard to digest and puts a load on your digestive system. Therefore, it is best if you opt for skimmed milk, which is much easier to digest.

Studies have shown that those who suffer from thyroid problems have also displayed low vitamin D levels, therefore, consider going for milk that has been fortified with vitamin D, to gain a dual benefit of your cup of milk.

2. Nuts

It is time to pack a small bag of some mixed nuts to snack with throughout your day. Studies show a link between eating nuts and its preventive power of hypothyroidism. One of the healthiest nuts you can eat for your thyroid health is walnuts. That is because they are rich in selenium. Low levels of selenium have been associated with those who suffered from thyroid diseases, especially hypothyroidism.

Another explorative study found selenium highly concentrated in the thyroid, more than any other organ in the body. Therefore, it was established that foods rich in selenium are thyroid friendly and helps it do its function.

Some studies claim that selenium helps detoxify the harmful product remains from the process of hormone production; therefore, keeping a clean environment from the thyroid to work optimally.

By eating nuts, especially Brazil nuts and walnuts, you are reducing the risks of suffering from goitre. Goitre typically arises from improper function of the thyroid gland, which can be prevented with adequate levels of selenium. Eating nuts also reduces the long-term effects of a damaged thyroid by increasing the levels of selenium in the body.

However, take care and take it slow, eating too many nuts can exceed the daily recommended levels of selenium.

3. Chicken

Another important nutrient is zinc. It helps the body to produce thyroid hormone. Chicken is a good source of zinc. In case you take too little amount of zinc, then you risk developing hypothyroidism due to a deficiency in thyroid hormone production. Zinc is needed for healthy thyroid function and also the reversal of some symptoms of thyroid hormone deficiency. For example, the hair loss due to hypothyroidism cannot be completely reversed with medication if the zinc stores in the body are not sufficient. Therefore, taking in food rich in zinc is necessary for your thyroid health and even the healing process, even if you are on medication.

Zinc also is needed for other important processes such as glucose regulation, and hair health. Make sure you get your daily recommended amount of zinc.

All in all, you probably get enough zinc through eating beef. However, it doesn't hurt to supplement this by eating chicken. Most meats are also a very good source of zinc.

4. Fish

On top of the fact that fish will increase your zinc levels, it can also help increase iodine in your body. They are a good source of selenium which is necessary for thyroid health. People who live in mountainous areas have a risk of developing a goitre. Therefore, to reduce this, you need to eat more fish, especially oily fish such as salmon, tuna, mackerel, etc.

Fish that is rich in omega 3 helps your body take off its cholesterol load and reduce the risk of heart diseases. When you suffer from a thyroid function imbalance, you suffer from imbalances in your metabolism and face an increased risk of heart diseases. The omega 3 in fatty fish can help you reduce inflammation and decrease the risk of developing heart diseases by reducing the level of circulating LDLs.

5. Eggs

Eggs are the best sources for selenium and iodine. Selenium will help activate the thyroid hormone. That is by converting your inactive T3 hormone into the active T4 hormone. It also acts as an antioxidant hence protecting the thyroid gland from damage by free radicals. One egg contains about 29% of your daily selenium requirements. It also provides about 8% of the daily iodine requirements, it might not be much but it adds up. You can have a thyroid friendly diet by including eggs.

Iodine, as explained earlier, helps in the proper function of the thyroid gland. It also reduces the chances of suffering from hypothyroidism.

6. Berries

Berries are a good source of vitamin D, selenium and iodine. Also, berries have a high concentration of antioxidants which is good for the thyroid gland. Therefore, if you are suffering from hypothyroidism, berries might be the best option for you.

Studies show that hypothyroidism patients have high levels of free radicals that can be counteracted by antioxidants in berries.

7. Soy

Consumption of soy for a healthy thyroid gland is still a huge debate. Some of the research done on soy suggests that it might have a negative effect especially if you have an iodine deficiency.

While other research suggests that unless you already have a problem with your thyroid, soy will not have any negative effect on it. All in all, unless you are taking a considerable amount of soy, then there's no need to worry.

8. Seaweed

Seaweed has high levels of iodine. However, the levels will greatly vary. But that doesn't mean you start eating sushi every single day. High levels of iodine in the body can also cause a lot of stress on your thyroid organ, hence causing harm.

9. Yogurt

Yogurt is also another great source of iodine. A major reason for this is because it's a live product containing culture. Most live culture yogurts contain iodine because of the cows the milk has come from are given iodine supplements and also the milking process typically involves using iodine-based cleaners.

10. Cauliflower

Cruciferous vegetables for instance cauliflower pack a lot of fiber which is good for your general health. However, you will need to be careful. In case you have an iodine deficiency, then consuming foods high in fiber might interfere with the production of thyroid hormone in your body. Therefore, you will need to limit your consumption of cauliflower and other cruciferous vegetables.

TOP SUPER FOOD RECIPES FOR THYROID HEALTH

SOY SLOW COOKED RIBS WITH SNAP PEAS

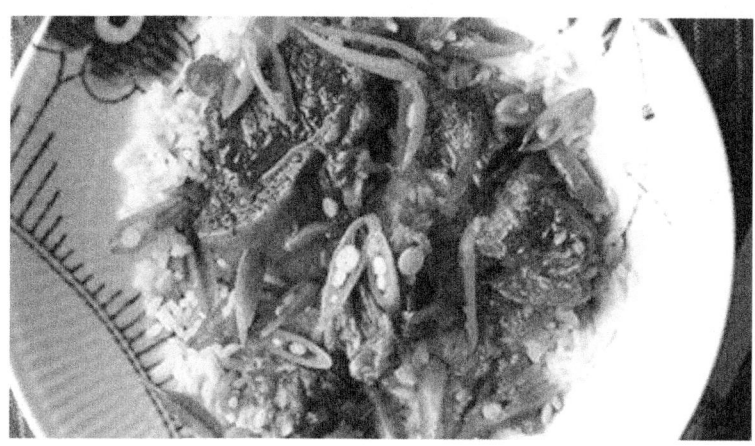

Total Prep Time: 8 hours and 30 Minutes

Serving: 6 servings

INGREDIENTS

- 1 medium onion, sliced
- 1/4 cup rice vinegar
- 4 cloves garlic, peeled and crushed
- 1/4 cup low-sodium soy sauce
- 2 tablespoons light brown sugar
- 1 teaspoon crushed red pepper
- 2 tablespoons chopped fresh ginger
- 3 pounds short ribs
- 2 cups white rice
- 1/2 pound snap peas, sliced

INSTRUCTIONS

1. Mix the onion, garlic, vinegar, ginger, soy sauce, sugar, red pepper, with ¼ cup water and add it to a suitable quart slow cooker.
2. Insert the beef in the mix and turn it to allow it to coat with the seasoning.
3. Insert the lid and cook until you feel the beef has become very tender. Do this on low heat for around 7 to 8 hours or on high heat for about 5 to 6 hours (this will shorten total recipe time). Skim off and discard most of the fat.

4. Before serving, cook and prepare the rice as per the package instructions.

5. Serve your slow-cooked tender soy beef over your rice. You can sprinkle sliced snap peas.

NUTRITIONAL INFORMATION

Calories 621

Fat 23g

Sat Fat 10g

Cholesterol 134mg

Sodium 416mg

Protein 48g

Carbohydrate 50g

Sugar 7g

Fiber 3g

Calcium 60mg

CAULIFLOWER RICE WITH SAUTÉD PEPPERS AND ONIONS

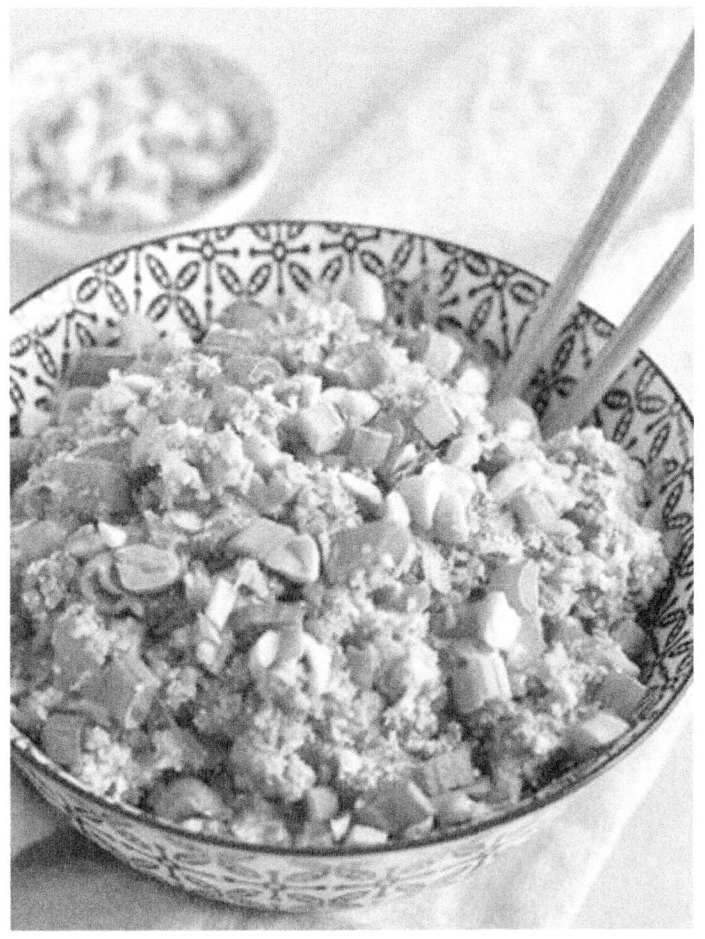

Total Prep Time: 15 Minutes

Serving: 4 servings

INGREDIENTS

- 1 head of cauliflower
- 2 green onions and fresh herbs of your choice, finely chopped
- 1 tablespoon of olive oil
- Kosher salt and black pepper to taste
- 1/2 of finely chopped bell pepper

INSTRUCTIONS

1. Prepare the cauliflower head by removing the leaves and separate the tough inner core using a sharp knife to make roughly chopped florets.
2. Add to food processer and pulse until you get a rice like consistency. You can cook all of it or freeze some for later.
3. Over a medium heat, in a suitable skillet, heat oil and sauté the chopped bell peppers and onions for few minutes.
4. Add the cauliflower and stir well then cover. Every once in a while, let the moisture out.

5. Let it cook for up to 5 minutes or until you feel that the cauliflower is tender and does not taste raw.

NUTRITIONAL INFORMATION:

Calories 820

Fat 5g

Sat Fat 1g

Cholesterol 1 mg

Sodium 200 mg

Protein 12 g

Carbohydrate 20 g

Sugar 7g

Fiber 13 g

Calcium 12%

CHICKEN FAJITA WITH CAULIFLOWER RICE

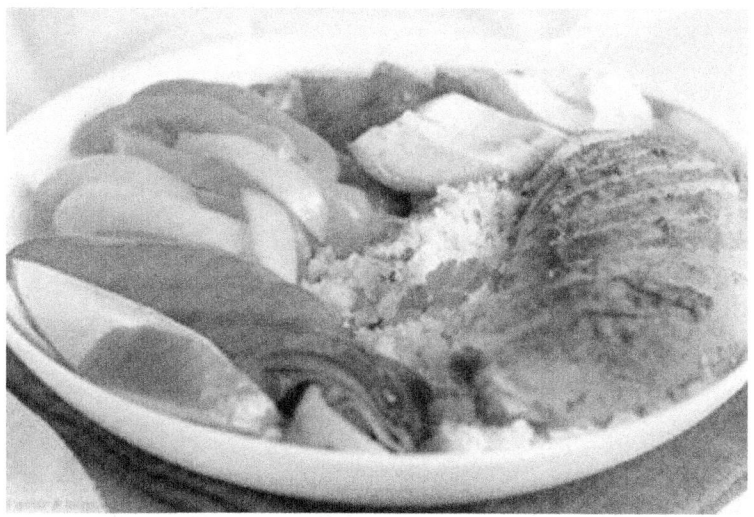

Total Prep Time: 30 Minutes

Serving: 2 servings

INGREDIENTS

- 2 large skinless boneless chicken breasts
- 1 tbsp oil (like grapeseed)
- 1 small red onion, sliced thinly
- 1 avocado, peeled, pit removed and sliced

- 3 bell peppers, red, orange, and yellow
- 1 cup fresh tomatoes, chopped
- 1 cup cauliflower rice

MARINADE

- 2 tbsp lime juice or lemon juice
- 2 tbsp olive oil
- 2 cloves garlic, minced
- 1/2 tsp sea salt
- 1/2 tsp ground cumin
- 1/2 tsp chili powder
- 1/2 tsp smoked paprika
- 1/4 cup chopped cilantro

INSTRUCTIONS

1. Prep your chicken breasts by cutting them into suitable thickness.
2. Mix the marinade ingredients together and add them to the chicken breasts. Let it marinate for 2-6 hours and no more than 8 hours.
3. Slice and chop the vegetables (onions, peppers and tomatoes).
4. Cook the cauliflower rice.

5. Heat oil in a suitable skillet to cook the chicken breasts, each side for about 5-7 minutes, (longer if breasts are thicker).

6. Meanwhile, sauté the peppers and onions.

7. Assemble the bowls with the cauliflower rice, peppers, onions and tomatoes.

8. Peel and slice avocado last to prevent browning. Add chicken to dish, drizzle with pan juices and serve immediately.

NUTRITIONAL INFORMATION

Calories 432kcal

Carbohydrates 24g

Protein 28g

Fat 25g

Saturated Fat 3g

Cholesterol 72mg

Sodium 755mg

Fiber 7g

Sugar 13g

Calcium 5.5%

KOREAN SEA WEED SOUP

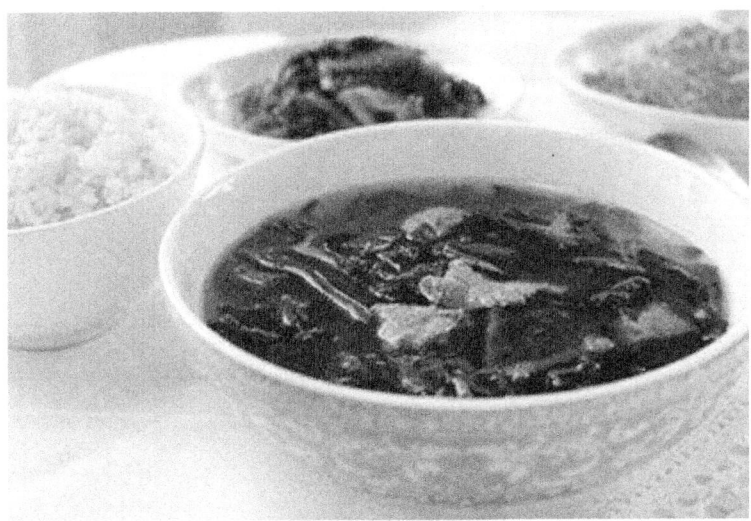

Total Prep Time: 45 Minutes

Yield: 4 servings

INGREDIENTS

- 1 (1 ounce) package dried brown seaweed
- 1/4 pound beef top sirloin, minced
- 2 teaspoons sesame oil
- 1 1/2 tablespoons soy sauce

- 1 teaspoon salt, or to taste
- 6 cups water
- 1 teaspoon minced garlic
- 1 (1 ounce) package dried brown seaweed
- 1/4 pound beef top sirloin, minced
- 2 teaspoons sesame oil
- 1 1/2 tablespoons soy sauce
- 1 teaspoon salt, or to taste
- 6 cups water
- 1 teaspoon minced garlic

INSTRUCTIONS

1. Soak the seaweed in water and cover it. Let it submerge until it becomes soft then drain and cut into two-inch pieces.
2. In a hot saucepan (medium heat); add the beef, 1 tbs of soy sauce sesame oil, and little salt, and let it cook for 2 minutes.
3. Add in seaweed and the remaining tbs of soy sauce and let it cook for 1 minute while stirring frequently.
4. Add two 2 cups of water and bring to a boil. Stir in garlic and remaining 4 cups water. let it boil then cover and reduce heat.

5. Simmer for 20 minutes. Season to taste with salt.

6. Soak the seaweed in water and cover it. Let it submerge until it becomes soft then drain and cut into two-inch pieces.

7. In a hot saucepan (medium heat); add the beef, 1 tbs of soy sauce sesame oil, and little salt, and let it cook for 2 minutes.

8. Add in seaweed and the remaining tbs of soy sauce and let it cook for 1 minute while stirring frequently.

9. Add two 2 cups of water and bring to a boil. Stir in garlic and remaining 4 cups water. let it boil then cover and reduce heat.

10. Simmer for 20 minutes. Season to taste with salt.

NUTRITIONAL INFORMATION

65 calories

3.7 g fat

1 g carbohydrates

0.8 Sugar

0.1 fiber

6.8 g protein

17 mg cholesterol

940 mg sodium

4% calcium

BLUEBERRY POPSICLES

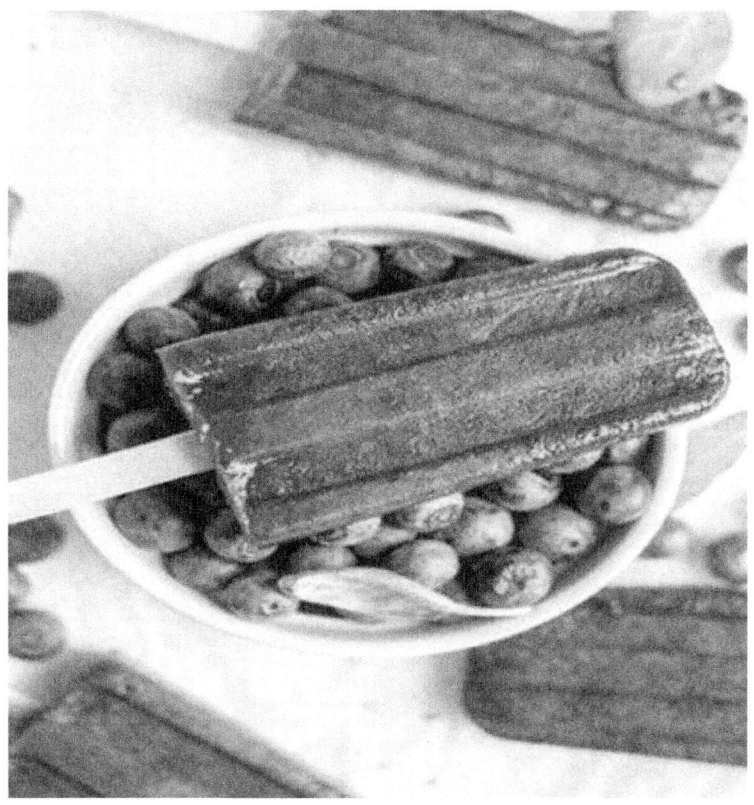

Total Prep Time: 8-10 hrs.

Yield: 4-6 Popsicles

INGREDIENTS

- 1 cup Vanilla yoghurt
- 2 Tablespoons Honey
- 2 cups blueberries

INSTRUCTIONS

1. Wash and add the blueberries in a blender/food processor.
2. Add yoghurt and honey.
3. Pour the mixture into Popsicle molds.
4. Put in the freezer for 4-6 hours or until frozen solid.

NUTRITIONAL INFORMATION

Calories 82

Total Fat 2.2g

Saturated fats 0

Sodium 21mg

Carbohydrates 12.3g

Sugar 8g

Fiber 3g

Protein 4.6g

WARM TURMERIC MILK

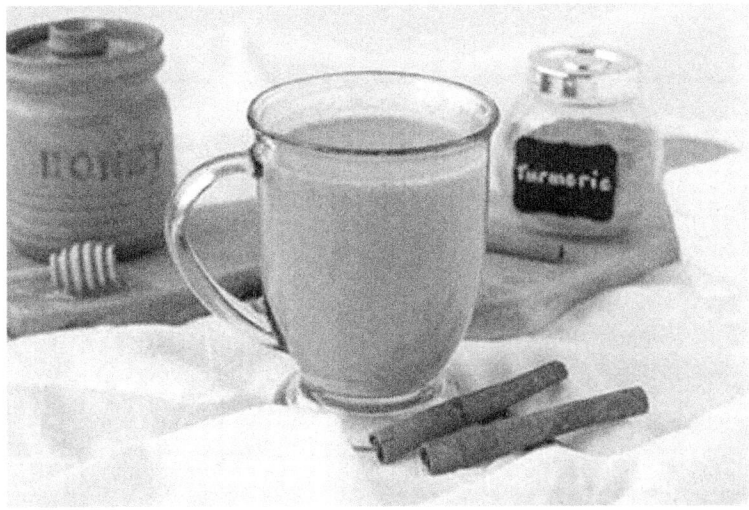

Total Prep Time: 6 minutes

Yield: 1 serving

INGREDIENTS

- 1 cup of milk
- 1 teaspoon of honey
- 1/4 teaspoon each of ground turmeric, cinnamon, ginger, and cardamom
- freshly ground black pepper

- 1 teaspoon coconut oil, optional

INSTRUCTIONS

1. In a suitable saucepan, heat the milk of your choice on low heat with the honey and optionally you can add coconut oil.
2. Let it almost boil, then turn off the heat.
3. Whisk in the spices until well blended. Pass through a fine mesh sieve.
4. Stir with a cinnamon stick.
5. Add some freshly ground pepper, stir again and serve.

NUTRITIONAL INFORMATION

Calories 95kcal

Carbohydrates 6g

Protein 1g

Fat 7g

Saturated Fat 3g

Sodium 325mg

Sugar 6g

Calcium 30%

FRESH YOGURT PARFAIT WITH BLUEBERRIES

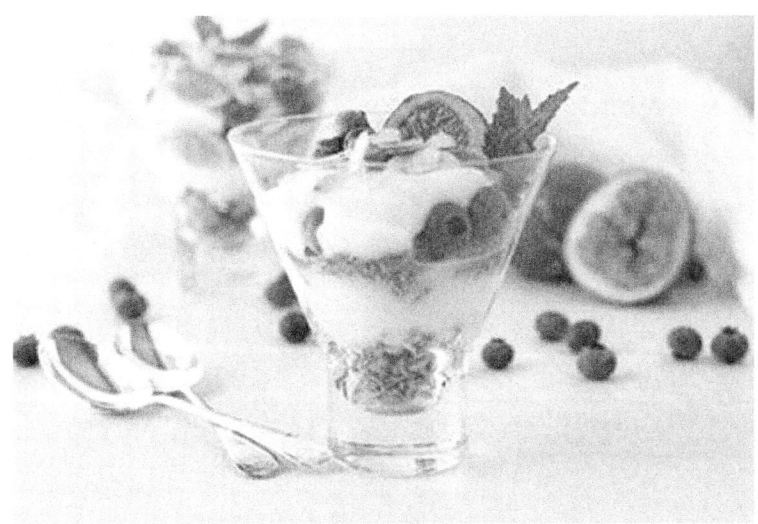

Total Prep Time: 3 minutes

Yield: 1 serving

INGREDIENTS

- 1 cup of yogurt
- 1/4 cup granola, it can be homemade or store-bought
- 1/4 cup blueberries, fresh or frozen

- 2 fresh figs, sliced
- 2 tsp honey or maple syrup
- 2 tbsp flaked toasted almonds

INSTRUCTIONS

1. Put the ingredients in a suitable glass or dessert cup in the following order: granola, then half the yogurt, then the fresh figs and blueberries, then the remaining yoghurt, and almonds.

2. Finally, garnish with a few blueberries, a slice of fig and a sprig of mint, if desired.

NUTRITIONAL INFORMATION

Calories 200

Fat 4 g

Sat Fat 10g

Cholesterol 0 mg

Sodium 50 mg

Protein 6 g

Carbohydrate 18 g

Sugar 7g

Fiber 6 g

Calcium 3%

STRAWBERRY RHUBARB PARFAIT

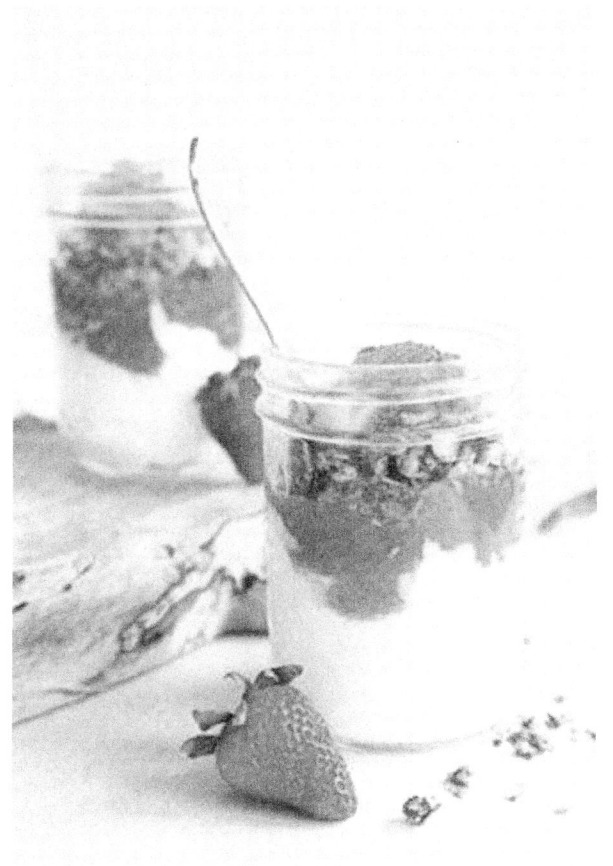

Total Prep Time: 5 minutes

Yield: 1 serving

INGREDIENTS

- 1 cup plain or vanilla Greek yoghurt or cultured coconut milk or yoghurt of your choice
- 1 tsp honey or maple syrup (optional)
- 1/4 cup rhubarb compote, see instructions below
- 2 strawberries, sliced thinly

INSTRUCTIONS

1. To make the rhubarb compote, add 4 cups chopped rhubarb stalks into a medium pot and 1/3 cup of water and 1/4 of cup maple syrup and stir.
2. Drop the heat when it starts to boil and let it simmer for 15-20 minutes until tender. Store in the fridge.
3. To make the parfait, mingle the yoghurt with either honey or maple syrup (optional). Add a little of it to a glass jar or any serving glass.
4. Add layers of rhubarb compote and freshly sliced strawberries.
5. Repeat the layers.
6. Garnish with a drizzle of honey, or a curl of rhubarb and chill or serve immediately.

NUTRITIONAL INFORMATION

Calories 150kcal

Carbohydrates 15g

Protein 20g

Cholesterol 10mg

Sodium 74mg

Fiber 1g

Sugar 12g

Calcium 24.6%

LOW CARB PANCAKES

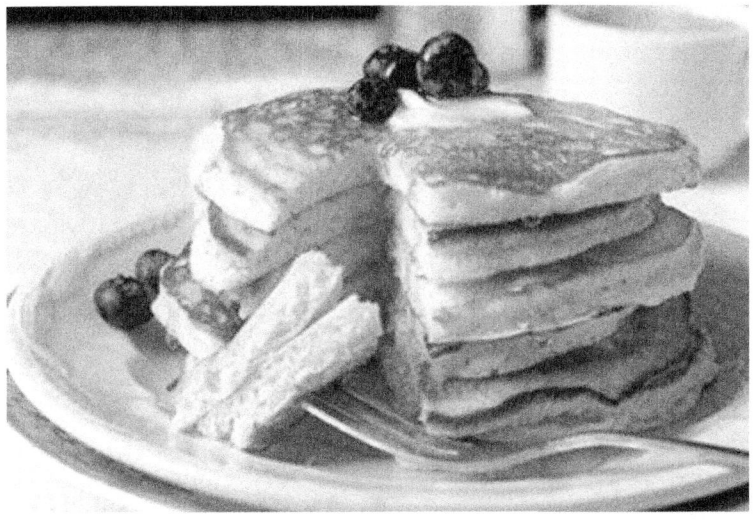

Total Prep Time: 5 minutes

Yield: 1 serving

INGREDIENTS

- 1 and half cups of cottage cheese
- 5 eggs
- 1/3 a cup of flour

INSTRUCTIONS

1. You want the cottage cheese to be a soft liquid so using your mixer, beat the cheese until it is mellow.
2. Then start by adding one egg and wait until it blends then add in the other one.
3. After the mixture evens out, start adding the flour bit by bit until the mixture becomes of even consistency. Now you have a pancake batter.
4. Pour in the amount that creates a thin film of liquid in your hot skillet and cook it for about 2 minutes then flip over to the other side and let it cook for 1-2 minutes on medium heat.

NUTRITIONAL INFORMATION

Calories 77

Total Fats 3

Saturated Fat 1 g

Sodium 45 mg

Carbohydrate 3 g

Sugars 2 g

Fiber 0

Protein 10 g

Viktoria McCartney

Calcium 3%

AVOCADO SHAKE

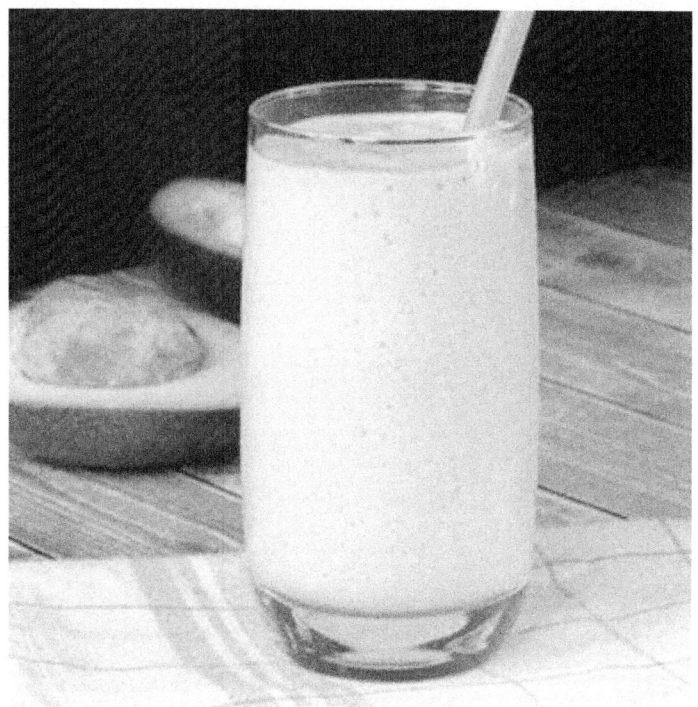

Total Prep Time: 5 minutes

Yield: 1 serving

INGREDIENTS

- One ripe avocado, pitted and peeled
- Five to 10 ice cubes: 5-10
- Quarter of cup of sweetened condensed milk: 1/4 cup

- Half a cup of cold milk: 1/2 cup

INSTRUCTIONS

In a blender take avocado, condensed milk, cold milk, ice cubes blend it smoothly.

NUTRITIONAL INFORMATION

540 Calories

Protein 6.7g

Total fat 1 g

Saturated 0

Carbohydrates 37g,

Sugar 32 g

Fiber 1 g

Cholesterol 24mg,

Sodium 97mg,

Calcium 12 %

BEST SUPER FOODS FOR LIVER HEALTH

The liver is one of the most powerful organs. That's because it performs a number of functions which include detoxification and break down of any toxins, protein production and clotting factors, storing excess glucose and controlling blood glucose level among others. Life is impossible without a liver. Meaning, you have to take care of its health.

That said, here are the best foods for your liver:

1. Avocado

Avocados are rich in healthy fat content that will ensure you have control of your weight. More to that, the fiber in avocados will also assist your digestive system. Avocado is basically a super food.

On top of controlling your weight, avocados contain glutathione which is a compound that helps the liver to get rid of toxins in its system. In addition, avocados are also able to cleanse your arteries.

2. Garlic

Is garlic a veggie or herb? Well, while you are still debating on this fact, studies have shown that garlic is good for your liver. Garlic contains a compound known as selenium which is a mineral that helps to detoxify the liver.

What's more, this great food is able to activate the liver enzymes that are responsible for flushing out toxins from your body. It also has allicin which helps to cleanse your liver. Studies have also shown that consumption of garlic will help you cut down on your weight.

3. Grapefruit

Grapefruit is also another great fruit that's helpful for your liver. It contains naringin which is an antioxidant that will naturally protect your liver through reducing inflammation and protecting the cells. That's not all!

This antioxidant will also reduce the occurrence of a harmful liver condition known as hepatic fibrosis. This condition leads to the excessive build-up of connective tissues within the liver.

Grapefruit also contain naringenin which decreases the levels of fat in the liver. Naringenin increases the production of enzymes associated with burning fats in the liver hence preventing any excessive accumulation of fats.

4. Fish

On top of the fact that fish is essentially helpful to your heart, it is also helpful to your liver. The omega-3 in fish is one of the healthy fats that reduce inflammation in your heart but also in your liver.

Studies have shown that omega-3 helps prevents fat build up, fight inflammation, improve insulin resistance and also keep a normal level of the enzymes in your liver. However, you need to ensure that you don't consume excess omega-3. The omega-3 to omega-6 ratio should be in check.

5. Berries

For instance, blueberries, are very powerful nutrient foods. Berries contain minerals, antioxidants (anthocyanins) and vitamins that give berries their distinct color. That said, anthocyanins have so far demonstrated anticarcinogenic, anti-inflammatory and antioxidant activities.

On top of that, these berries can also protect your liver from damage. Several studies have shown that berry juice or extract also keep your liver healthy. They are able to boost your immune response and also lower inflammation.

6. Olive Oil

Besides the fact that olive oil is good for your heart, it can also prove to be helpful for your liver.

Additionally, olive oil helps to reduce the fat levels in the liver. It also helps increase blood flow around your entire body. More to that, olive oil also helps to improve the levels of liver enzymes.

7. Tea

Tea is widely known for its health benefits. Studies have also shown that tea is particularly beneficial to your liver. That's because both the black and green tea are able to improve enzyme levels as well as reduce the levels of fat in the liver. It is rich in antioxidants which ease the work of the liver and helps it in detoxifying.

8. Leafy vegetables

Leafy green vegetables contain high amounts of minerals. Some of these minerals include potassium, magnesium and manganese. Also, the chlorophyll found in leafy veggies helps to purify the blood.

On top of that, chlorophyll assists in neutralizing heavy metals, pesticides and toxic chemicals which might be a burden to the liver. Some of these green veggies include kale, spinach, collards among others.

9. Eggs

Organic eggs are a good source of nutrients that are important to the liver. They contain glutathione, sulphur compound and methylation elements. What's more, they contain omega-3, vitamin D and other healthy saturated fats that maintain a healthy and strong cell membrane. Eggs are also quite delicious as a morning breakfast.

10. Coffee

Finally, coffee is one of the best beverages for a healthy liver. Coffee is able to protect your liver from diseases. Drinking coffee will help you reduce risks of suffering from liver cancer. On top of that, coffee is able to reduce inflammation and effects of other liver diseases.

TOP SUPER FOOD RECIPES FOR LIVER HEALTH

AVOCADO WRAPS

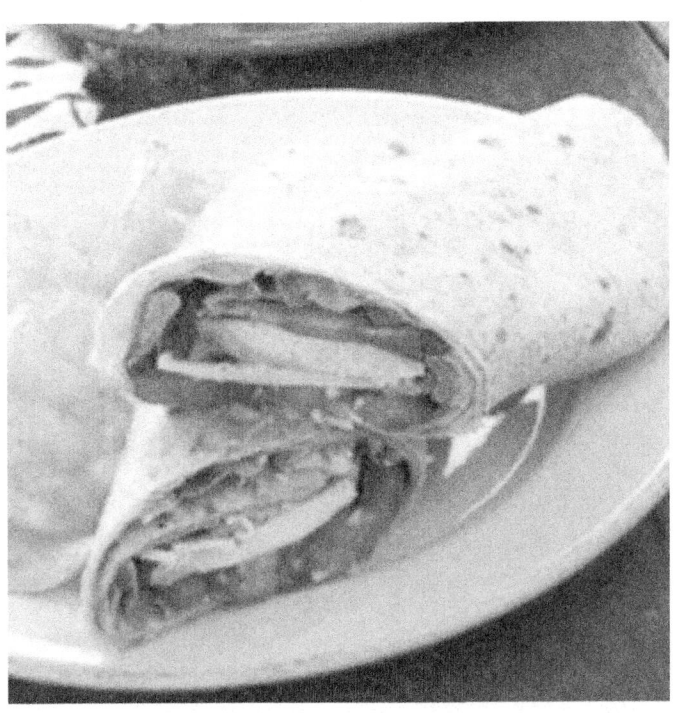

Total Prep Time: 10 minutes

Yield: 1 serving

INGREDIENTS

- 1/2 medium ripe avocado, peeled and thinly sliced
- 1/2 medium thinly sliced tomato
- 1 flavored tortilla
- 1 tablespoon shredded Parmesan cheese
- 1 lettuce leaf
- 1/8 teaspoon garlic powder
- Salt according to taste.
- pepper according to taste

INSTRUCTIONS

1. In a bowl, mash avocado add garlic powder, salt and pepper.
2. Now spread the mix over to tortillas.
3. Layer with lettuce, tomato and remaining avocado.
4. Sprinkle with cheese, roll up.
5. Serve immediately.

NUTRITIONAL INFORMATION

176 calories

8g fat

3g saturated fat

2mg cholesterol

228mg sodium

22g carbohydrate

2g sugars

4g fiber

5g protein

8% calcium

GARLIC BUTTER

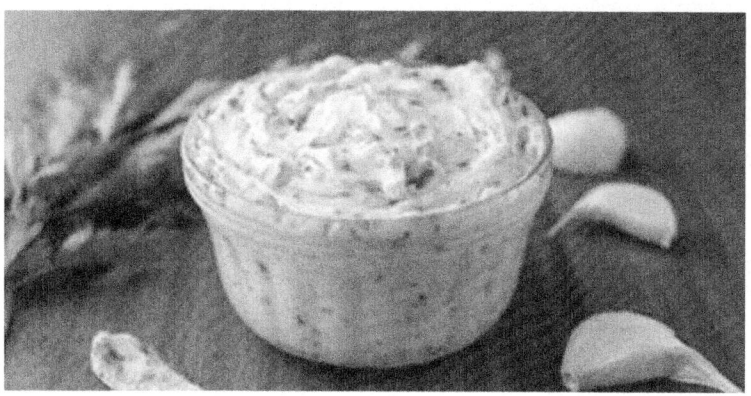

Total Preparation Time: 2 minutes

Yield: 2 servings

INGREDIENTS

- 1 lb. unsalted butter (Room temperature)
- 2 tablespoons fresh chopped parsley
- Salt according to taste
- 5 large peeled garlic cloves

INSTRUCTIONS

1. Put all ingredients in a bowl and mix it well.
2. Garlic Butter is ready. Chill or freeze until needed.

NUTRITIONAL INFORMATION

216 Calories

23g Fat

2 g Saturated

0.2 mg cholesterol

260 mg sodium

3g Carbohydrates

1g Sugar

2g Fiber

1 g Protein

10% Calcium

GARLIC CROUTONS

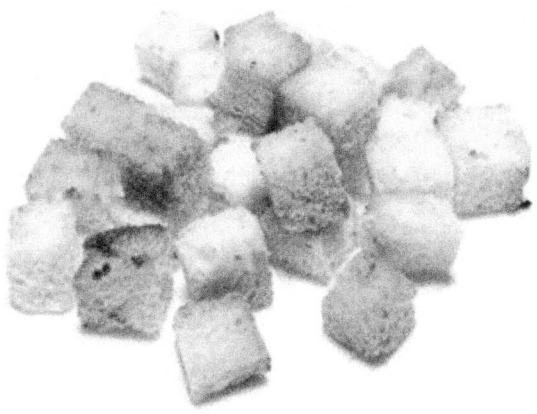

Total Preparation Time: 25 minutes

Yield: 2 servings

INGREDIENTS

- 3 slices white bread, cut into1/4-inch cubes
- 3 tablespoons virgin olive oil
- 2 garlic cloves

INSTRUCTIONS

1 Preheat oven to 350°F.

2 In a bowl, mix garlic, salt, olive oil. Pour this mixture to bread cubes. Toss to coat. Spread the bread on a baking sheet.

3 In a suitable pan, melt the butter over medium heat. Stir in garlic; cook and stir for 1 minute. Add bread cubes and toss to coat. Spread on a baking sheet.

4 Bake for 15 minutes, or until it is slightly browned crisp and dry. Check frequently to prevent burning.

NUTRITIONAL INFORMATION

89 calories

7.8 g fat

2 g saturated fats

4.2 g carbohydrates

2 g sugars

1 g fiber

0.9 g protein

20 mg cholesterol

101 mg sodium

GRAPEFRUIT MOJITO

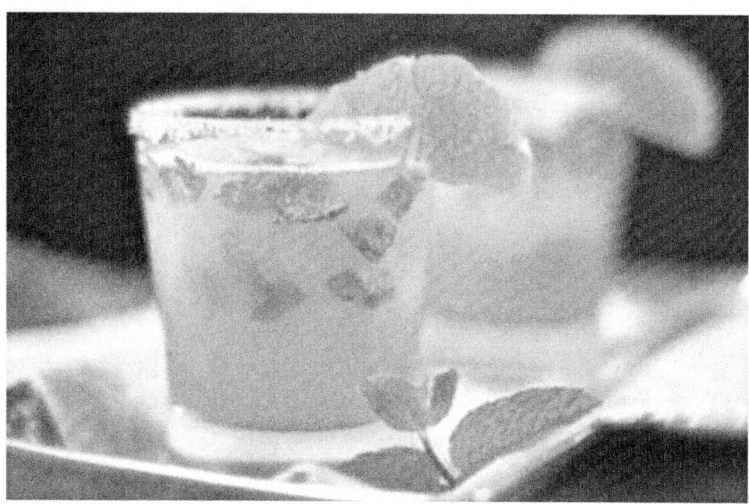

Total Preparation Time: 5 minutes

Yield: 2 servings

INGREDIENTS

- Zest and juice (3 to 4 tablespoons) of 1/2 grapefruit
- 1 piece of grapefruit wedge (for decoration)
- 2 tablespoons sugar crushed
- Ice
- Champagne or soda

- 2 tablespoons of fresh lime juice
- 20 fresh mint leaves, 3-4 mints for garnishing
- 1-2 ounces white rum

INSTRUCTIONS

1. In a shaker, pour lime juice, sugar, mint leaves and grapefruit zest.
2. Stir it with spoon until the sugar melts.
3. Add the grapefruit juice and rum.
4. Fill with ice and shake.
5. Strain into 2 glasses and top off with the club soda or champagne.
6. Garnish with a mint and grapefruit wedge in each glass.

NUTRITIONAL INFORMATION

Calories 320

Total Fat 0.4gm

Saturated 0

Cholesterol 0

Carbohydrate 84.8g

Sugar 32 g

Fiber 9 g

Protein 1.9g

Calcium 12 %

HOT SPICED GREEN TEA

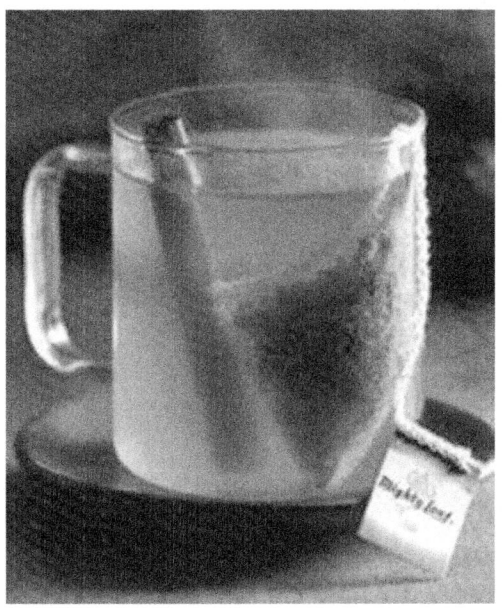

Total Preparation Time: 5 minutes

Yield: 1 servings

INGREDIENTS

- 1 Cinnamon stick
- 2 green tea bags
- 2 cardamom pods

- 2 boiling water
- 1 tablespoon honey
- ¼ teaspoon minced ginger
- ½ teaspoon grated lemon zest

INSTRUCTIONS

1. In a bowl, combine add all the ingredients except honey.
2. Cover it for 5 minutes.
3. Strain, tea and add honey into tea.
4. Serve hot.

NUTRITIONAL INFORMATION

Calorie 33

Carbohydrates 9g

Total Fat 0.0 gm

Saturated 0

Cholesterol 0

Sugar 3 g

Fiber 0.1 g

Protein 0.1 g

Calcium 1 %

CHICKEN SOUP

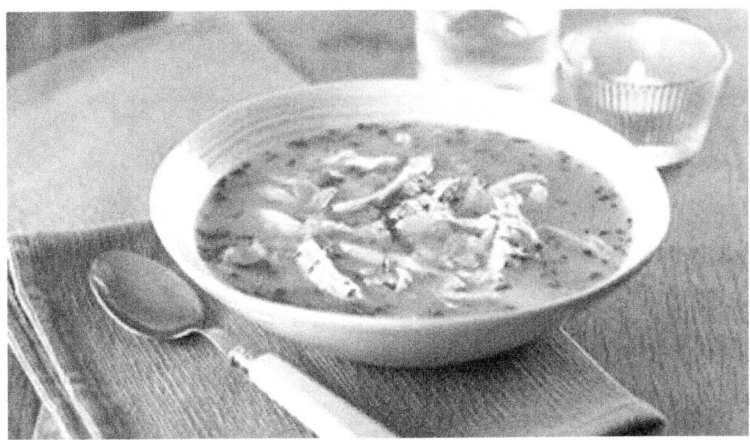

Total Preparation Time: 25 minutes

Yield: 8 servings

INGREDIENTS

- 8 cups water
- medium onions
- garlic crushed
- Salt to taste
- 4 pounds whole chicken
- 2 celery stalks

- medium sliced carrots

INSTRUCTIONS

1 Take chicken, 1 tablespoon salt and water in a pot.

2 Boil all these.

3 Add onions, garlic and celery.

4 Reduce heat, cover it partially for half an hour after that remove breast and kept it aside.

5 Add carrots in it. Simmer, partially covered, for 40 minutes.

6 Remove remaining chicken and wings and bones. Cut into bite-size pieces.

7 Stir in desired amount of chicken; season with salt.

8 Serve hot.

NUTRITIONAL INFORMATION

Calorie 36

Total carbs 1.2 g

Sugar 1 g

Fiber 0.2

Protein 2.5g

Cholesterol 105 mg

Sodium 143 mg

Calcium 4 %

GINGER BREAD COFFEE

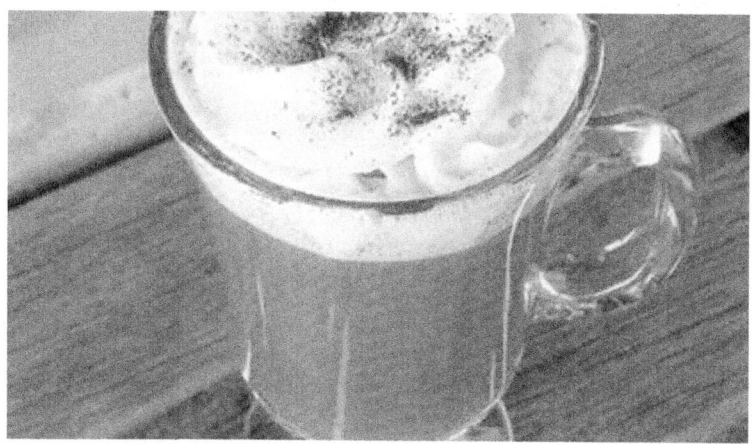

Total Preparation Time: 5 minutes

Yield: 1 serving

INGREDIENTS

- 1/2 cup molasses
- 1/4 cup brown sugar
- 1/2 teaspoon baking soda
- 1 teaspoon ground ginger
- 3/4 teaspoon ground cinnamon
- 6 cups hot brewed coffee

- 1 cup half-and-half cream
- 1 teaspoon ground cloves
- 1 1/2 cups sweetened whipped cream

INSTRUCTIONS

1. In a suitable bowl, blend together the molasses, brown sugar, ginger, baking soda, and cinnamon until well mixed.
2. Cover the mix and let it refrigerate for at least 10 minutes.
3. Add around a 1/4 cup of coffee to each cup.
4. Add round a tablespoon of the spice mixture until dissolved.
5. Fill a cup to near an inch of the top with coffee.
6. Add half and half cream to taste.
7. Garnish with whipped cream as desired.

NUTRITIONAL INFORMATION

198 calories

8.1 g fat

30.6 g carbohydrates

23 g sugar

5 g fiber

2 g protein

26 mg cholesterol

158 mg sodium

6% Calcium

GARNISHED FISH

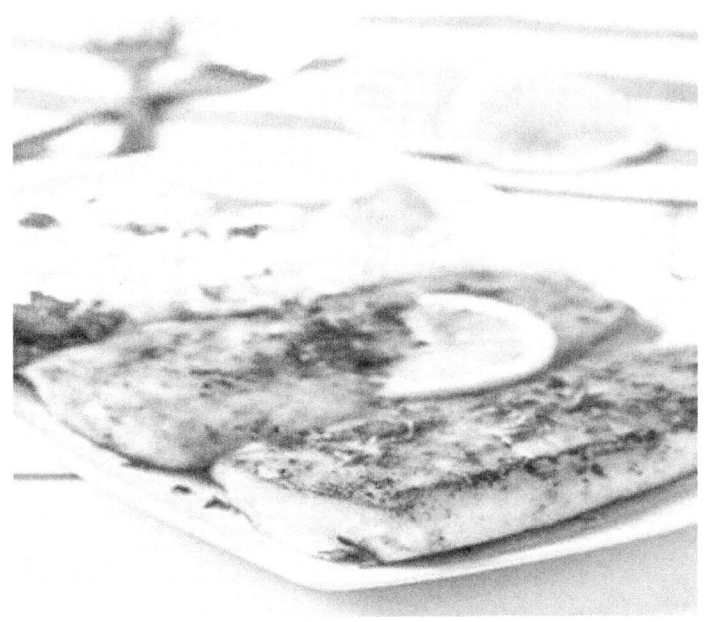

Total Preparation Time: 20 minutes

Yield: 4 servings

INGREDIENTS

- firm white fish fillets, 1-inch thick.
- 3 TB melted butter (I use salted)
- 1 tsp paprika

- Juice and zest from 1 medium lemon
- 1 tsp garlic powder
- 1 tsp onion powder
- 3 TB olive oil
- 1 tsp kosher salt or to taste
- Freshly chopped basil or some parsley leaves (optional)
- 1/4 tsp freshly ground black pepper
- Extra lemon slices for serving

INSTRUCTIONS

1. Dry any moisture from fish fillets using paper towels and keep fish aside.
2. Using a suitable a bowl, mix the melted butter with the lemon juice and the lemon zest, and add 1/2 tsp of kosher salt. Don't forget to stir to blend well.
3. In another bowl, put the remaining 1/2 tsp kosher salt with the paprika, garlic powder, onion powder, and the black pepper. Mix and evenly apply the spice mixture to both the sides of fish fillets to season.
4. In a suitable non-stick pan, over medium-high heat, heat the olive oil to cook the fish fillets. Don't overcrowd to allow browning.

5. Slowly sprinkle some of the lemon butter sauce on the fish as you are cooking but save some for dressing.

6. Don't overcook the fish.

7. Serve your fish with the rest of the prepped lemon butter sauce or add basil or parsley, and lemon wedges on top for decorations.

NUTRITIONAL INFORMATION

Calorie 48

Fats 8 g

Saturated 0.1

Carbohydrates 1.1 g

Sugar 0.5 g

Fiber 0.6 g

Protein 3.5g

Cholesterol 85 mg

Sodium 143 mg

Calcium 4.2 %

MIXED BEAN SALAD WITH OLIVE OIL DRESSING

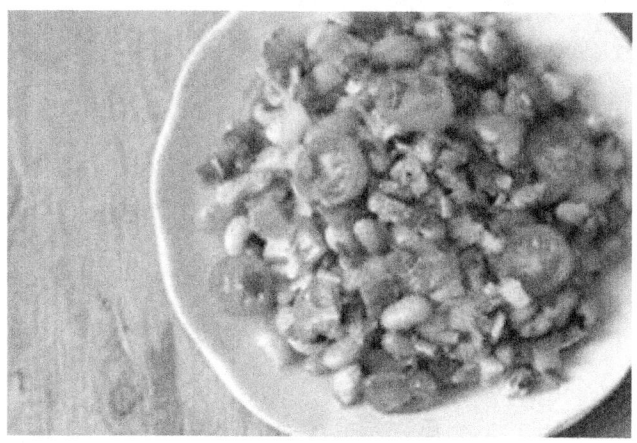

Total Preparation Time: 1 hour 15 minutes

Yield: 6 servings

INGREDIENTS

- ½ can black beans rinsed and drained
- ½ can cannellini beans drained and rinsed
- ½ can kidney beans, drained
- ½ tablespoon lemon juice
- 1 tablespoon white sugar

- 1 clove crushed garlic
- ½ red bell pepper, chopped
- 1/2 green bell pepper, chopped
- 1/2 tablespoon salt
- ½ package frozen corn kernels
- 1/4 tablespoon ground cumin
- 1/8 cup chopped fresh cilantro
- 1/2 red onion, chopped
- 1/4 cup olive oil
- 1/2 dash hot pepper sauce
- ¼ tablespoon ground black pepper
- ¼ teaspoon chili powder
- ¼ cup red wine vinegar
- 1 tablespoon fresh lime juice

INSTRUCTIONS

1. In a bowl, stir olive oil, garlic, lime-juice, sugar, salt, garlic, black pepper, red wine vinegar, cilantro, cumin, hot sauce and chili powder.
2. In a bowl, add red onion, beans, bell peppers and frozen corn.
3. Mix oil dressing with vegetables, salad is ready!
4. Serve cold.

NUTRITIONAL INFORMATION

334 calories

Carbohydrates 41.5g

Sugars 9

Fiber 23

Fat 14.5g

Saturated fats 1 g

Protein 11 g

Sodium 1160 mg

Calcium 8%

VIENNEXICAN COFFEE

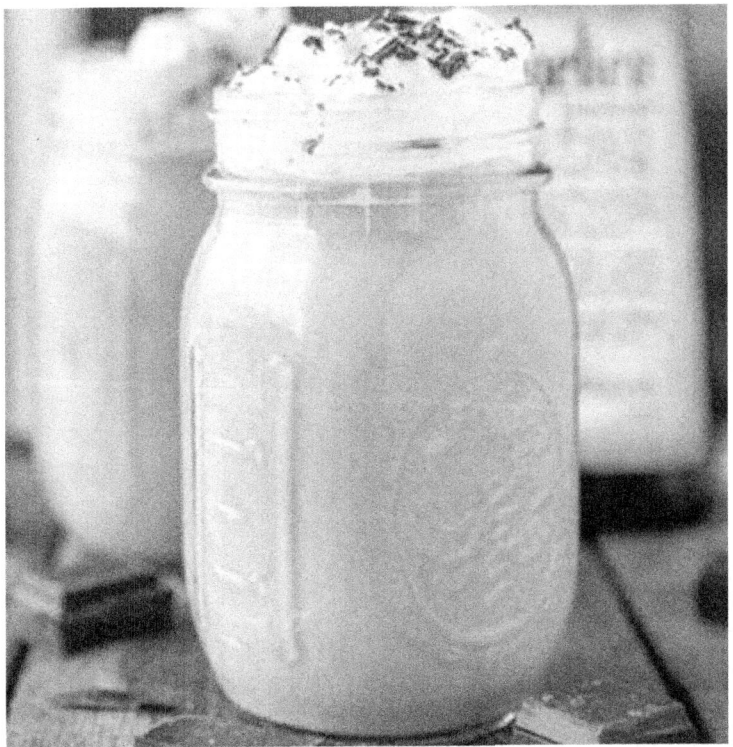

Total Preparation Time: 5 minutes

Yield: 1 serving

INGREDIENTS

- 1 teaspoon cocoa powder
- 1 tablespoon heavy whipping cream
- tablespoons whole milk
- 1 cup hot brewed coffee
- 1 1/2 teaspoons brown sugar
- 1/2 teaspoon orange extract
- 1/2 teaspoon vanilla extract
- 1/2 teaspoon ground cinnamon
- 1/8 teaspoon ground nutmeg

INSTRUCTIONS

1. Stir all the ingredients in a pitcher until smooth.
2. Serve chill coffee.

NUTRITIONAL INFORMATION

Calories 129

Fat 7.5g

Saturated fats 0.1 g

Sodium 32mg

Carbohydrate 11.9g

Sugars 8 g

Fiber 0.1 g

Protein 2.5 g

Calcium 2 %

BEST SUPER FOODS FOR SKIN AND HAIR

Are you looking for a natural way to achieve that glowing skin and healthy hair? Well, this chapter is just what you need. You've probably heard this a million times, but again, I'd say that you really are what you eat.

Therefore, you can easily influence your looks by consuming certain foods. In that case, below is a list of foods that you need to get that desired glow on.

1. Fatty Fish

Fatty fish is one of the major sources of omega-3 fats. These omega-3 fats are known to have high anti-inflammatory effects. In that case, it offers incredible beauty benefits such as healthy hair strands and glowing skin.

In addition to that, the fatty fish provides a carotenoid known as astaxanthin. This helps with reducing wrinkles as well as any other signs of ageing. Besides that, fatty fish is also a great source of selenium, proteins, Vitamins D3 and B which are all nutrients linked to healthy and strong hair growth.

The omega 3 in fatty fish helps to fortify and thicken the skin. This increases the integrity of the cell membranes. When you have good skin integrity, that means you have better protection against ultra violet rays and the escape of moisture from your skin.

Omega 3 fatty acid also helps to retain water in your skin, this causes your skin to retain moisture and softness. That will give you a soft and nourished skin and help you get rid of dry scaly skin.

2. Eggs

Also, another great source of proteins as well as biotin. These are the two major nutrients that contribute to healthy hair growth. Hair follicles are majorly made of proteins; hence there is a need for adequate proteins in your diet.

On the other hand, biotin helps with the production of the hair protein known as keratin. All in all, eggs make a great source for selenium and zinc; hence one of the top of the chart foods for optimal hair growth. They are also rich in vitamin E which is optimum for your hair and skin health.

3. Green Tea

Green tea contains catechin which is a protective antioxidant for anti-ageing. in that case, the catechin helps to prevent the skin from damage that could be caused by free radicals. The antioxidant effect also soothes any irritated or inflamed skin. This will leave you with a clear and radiant skin. The anti-inflammatory properties of green tea also helps against acne out breaks.

Green tea also has anti-aging properties by promoting rapid cell turnover, that means quick bye-bye to old skin and hello new, fresh, radiant youthful skin. To top it all, green tea could help improve the moisture levels of the skin, its plumpness and its elasticity. It also helps stimulate the hair follicles in your scalp to grow more hair, faster.

4. Dark Chocolate

You might end up making dark chocolate your new best friend after reading this. Dark chocolate contains cocoa. Cocoa has phenomenal effects on the skin, and this is a good reason to eat chocolate. Cocoa is high in antioxidants hence could help you achieve more hydrated and plumper skin. Also, chocolate is high in flavanols that contribute to healthier blood flow.

In that case, more nutrients, as well as oxygen, are transported to the skin. This will, in turn, improve the general appearance of the skin. It is also rich in minerals like zinc which improve your skin cell turnover and growth cycles. Dark chocolate is the key to a youthful and younger looking healthy skin.

5. Avocados

Avocados are rich in healthy fats which influence the general functioning of the body. This includes the general well-being of the skin too. In that, the skin remains well moisturized and flexible.

Also, avocados make an excellent source for vitamin E. That is because it helps with skin healing as well as moisturizing the skin. The fats present in avocados keep the skin soft and the hair in a good condition.

6. Carrots

Carrots are a known great source of beta carotene which in the body gets converted to vitamin A. This is an essential vitamin in the body that helps to maintain the firmness of the skin.

Also, beta-carotene helps to prevent the skin from damage. At the same time, it ensures that you have a healthy scalp and strong shiny hair.

7. Pomegranates

Pomegranates are rich in punicalagins which is a very powerful anti-oxidant. Punicalagins have strong anti-inflammatory as well as anti-oxidant effects.

These two properties help to protect the skin against free radical damage. This is because free radical damage is one of the major contributors to skin ageing.

8. Quinoa

This is another great food source that helps you improve and maintain healthy skin and hair all at the same time. Quinoa is rich in vitamins B, zinc, fiber and iron.

Zinc is the most important nutrient as it helps with cell growth in the body. In that case, it is essential in boosting growth as well as repair of hair follicles.

9. Blueberries

Like most berries, blueberries are packed with high levels of flavonoids. Flavonoids is a type of antioxidant compound that protects your skin from ageing.

What's more, blueberries are also an excellent source of vitamin C which is essential for healthy collagen formation. This makes blueberries the best food if you want to maintain a healthy skin and hair.

10. Kale

Kales is one of the most important sources of iron. More to that, it also helps to ensure a smooth blood flow to your skin and hair since this flow is dependent on the presence of iron. Additionally, kale is also a good source of vitamins A, E and C which will boost your immunity.

Top Super food Recipes for Skin and Hair

KALE WITH WHITE BEANS

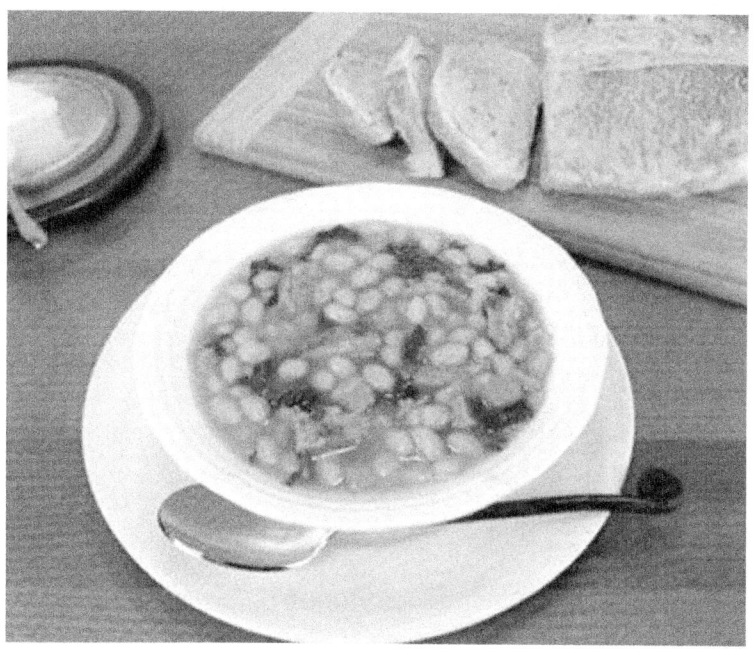

Total Prep Time: 30 Minutes

Yield: 2 servings

INGREDIENTS

- 1 cup chopped raw kale
- ½ tablespoon olive oil
- 2 small garlic cloves
- 2 tablespoon yellow chopped onion
- ½ cup chicken or vegetable broth
- 2-ounces white beans
- ½ chopped tomato
- 1 tablespoon chopped parsley
- Salt, pepper and Italian herb seasoning to taste

INSTRUCTIONS

1. In a sauce pan heat oil sauté onion and garlic and kale until wilted.
2. Add 1.5-ounce beans, ¼ broth, tomato, salt, pepper and herbs.
3. Cook for 5 mins.
4. In a bender blend the remaining broth and beans until smooth.
5. Pour this mix into soup so that the soup will thicken.

6. Garnish the soup with parsley.

NUTRITIONAL INFORMATION

Calories 182

Fat 2.5 g

Saturated fats 1 g

Cholesterol 0 mg

Sodium 220 mg

Protein 11 g

Carbohydrates; 31 g

Sugar 5 g

Fiber 12 g

Protein 11 g

Calcium 6.4%

AVOCADO ICE CREAM

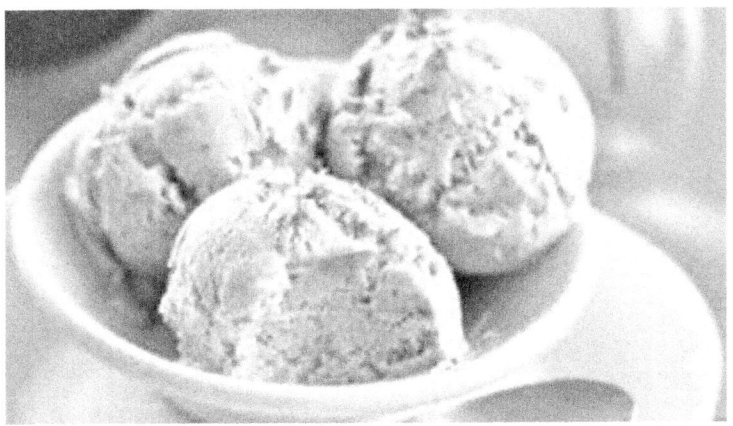

Total Prep Time: 35 Minutes

Yield: 6 servings

INGREDIENTS

- One 8-ounce avocado pitted and peeled
- 2 tablespoons lemon juice
- Pinch fine salt
- One 14-ounce can sweetened condensed milk
- 2 cups cold heavy cream

INSTRUCTIONS

1. In a blender take an avocado, milk, lemon juice and salt, blend it until smooth.
2. On a medium speed, start by whipping the heavy cream until firm peaks form.
3. With a spatula, fold 1 cup of the whipped cream into the avocado puree.
4. When it is well blended, fold the lightened mixture back into the whipped cream.
5. Pour the mixture into the freezer, until it is frozen.
6. Ice- cream is ready.

NUTRITIONAL INFORMATION

220 Calories

Carbohydrate 29 g

Sugar 22 g

Fat 10 g

Saturated fats 2g

Protein 3g

Sodium 60mg

Cholesterol 30mg

Viktoria McCartney

Calcium 7%

POMEGRANATE FETA SALAD WITH LEMON DIJON VINAIGRETTE

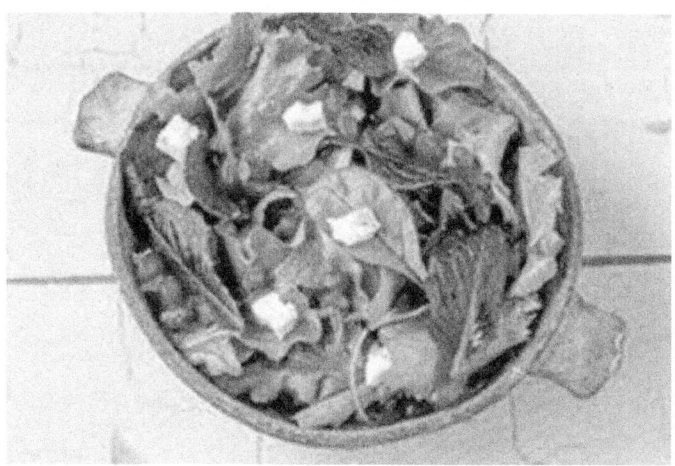

Total Prep Time: 15 Minutes

Yield: 5 servings

INGREDIENTS

- 10 ounces mixed baby greens
- 1 separated seeds pomegranate
- 8-ounce package crumbled cheese feta
- 1 teaspoon Dijon mustard

- 3 tablespoons red wine vinegar
- Salt and pepper to taste
- 1 lemon juiced and zested
- 3 tablespoon olive oil
- 2 lettuce

INSTRUCTIONS

1. Place the lettuce, pomegranate seeds and cheese into a suitable bowl.
2. Add the lemon juice olive oil, and zest, mustard, salt, and pepper, vinegar in a separate bowl.
3. Pour this to the salad and mix to let it coat with the dressing mix.

NUTRITIONAL INFORMATION

Calories 230

Carbohydrates 12 g

Sugar 2 g

Fiber 8 g

Fat 18 g

Saturated fats 2g

Protein 7.8g

Cholesterol 40 mg

Sodium 549 mg

Calcium 4.2 %

WOJABI

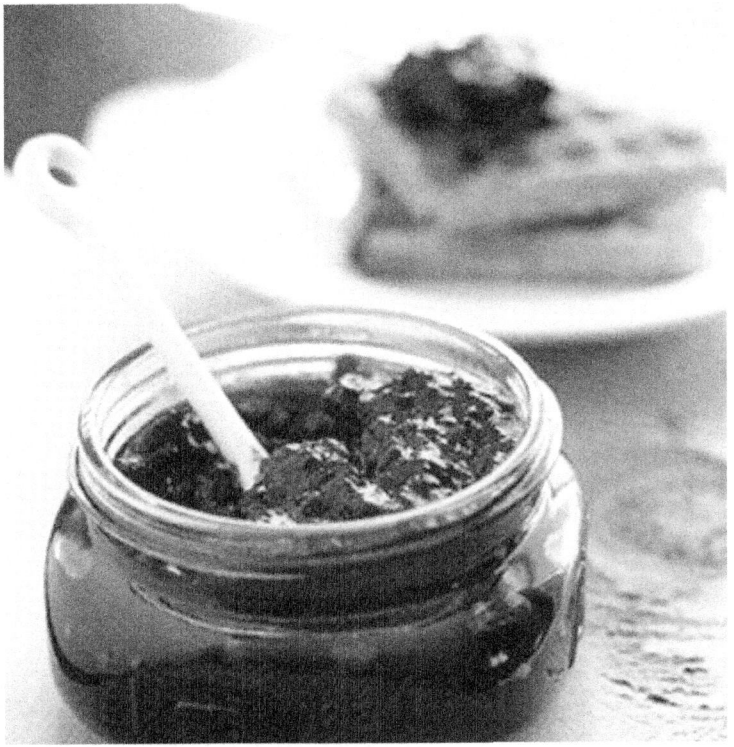

Total Prep Time: 1 hour 30 Minutes

Yield: 6 servings

INGREDIENTS

- 1 ½ cups Blueberries, Raspberries or Strawberries
- 2 Tablespoons of Honey
- 1 cup of water

INSTRUCTIONS

1 Mash the berries in a mixing bowl.

2 Add water to a pan and let it boil, pour the mashed berries into it.

3 Cook for one hr. on a low heat.

4 Add honey.

5 Stir gently to combine and constantly until you have the desired consistency.

NUTRITIONAL INFORMATION

Calories 13

Sugar 2 g

Carbohydrates 3g

Fiber 0.5 g

Sodium 52 mg

Cholesterol 0.1

Viktoria McCartney

Calcium 4%

GARLIC ROASTED CARROTS

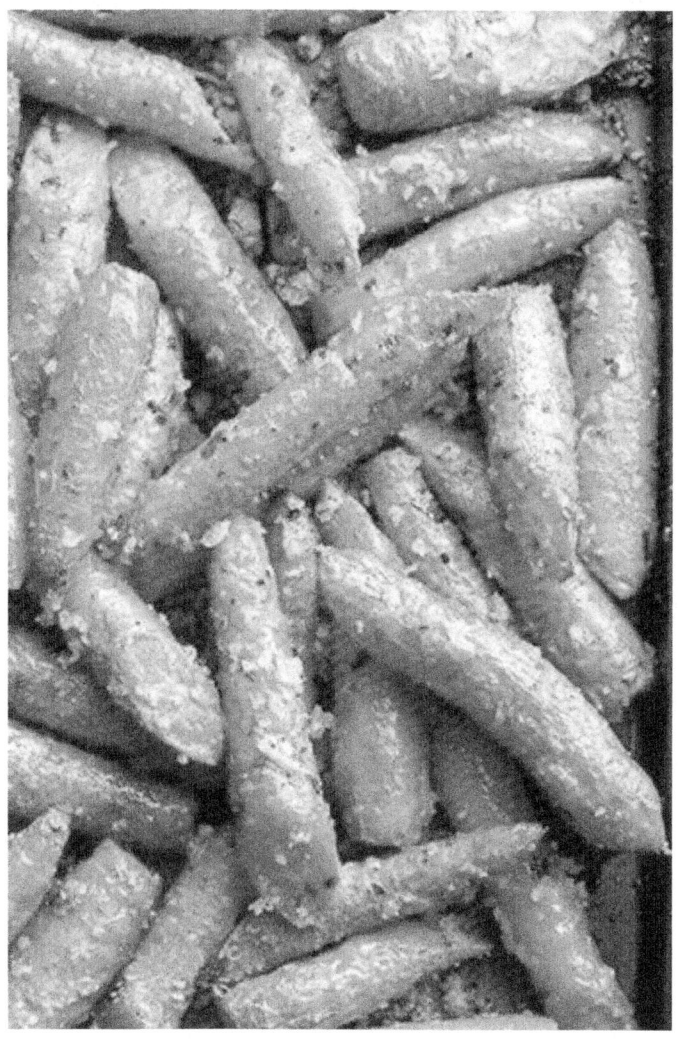

Total Prep Time: 30 Minutes

Yield: 4 servings

INGREDIENTS

- 2 pounds (1kg) carrots, washed and halved
- 1/4 cup grated parmesan cheese
- 1/4 cup olive oil
- Salt and pepper, to taste
- 4 large cloves garlic, minced (or 1 tablespoon minced garlic)
- 2 tablespoons of bread crumbs
- Fresh chopped parsley, optional

INSTRUCTIONS

1. Preheat your oven to (400°F) and prepare a sprayed baking sheet with cooking oil.
2. Arrange the carrots on the baking sheet.
3. Add some olive oil, next, add the garlic and parmesan cheese, and sprinkle the bread crumbs, salt and pepper.
4. Mix all ingredients well to cover the carrots fully.
5. Spread the carrots out evenly and bake for 25 minutes while turning half time.

6. Serve instantly; you can also top it with fresh parsley if you want.

NUTRITIONAL INFORMATION

Calorie 95

Total fat 3 g

Saturated fats 0.1

Sodium 344mg

Carbohydrates16g

Sugar 4 g

Fiber 9 g

Calcium2.5%

HOME MADE DARK CHOCOLATE

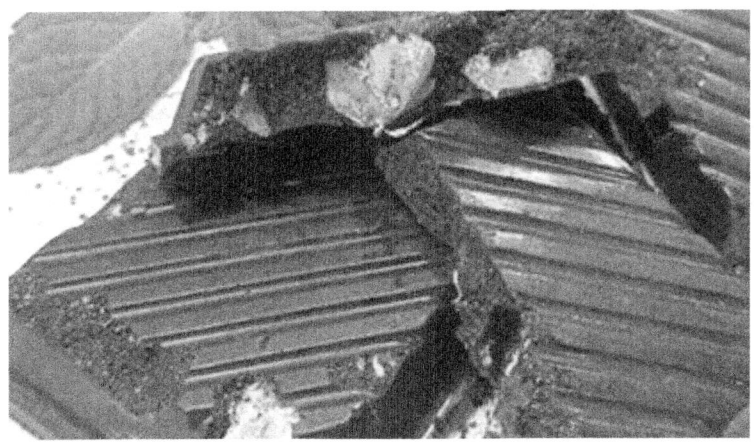

Total Prep Time: 15 Minutes

Yield: 4 servings

INGREDIENTS

- 1/2 cup coconut oil
- 1/2 cup cocoa powder
- 3 tablespoons honey
- 1/2 teaspoon vanilla extract

INSTRUCTIONS

1. Slowly allow the coconut oil to melt in a saucepan by applying medium-low heat.
2. Add in cocoa powder, some honey, and a pinch of vanilla extract into the melted oil until it is all well blended.
3. Pour mixture into a candy mold.
4. Refrigerate until chilled, about 1 hour.

NUTRITIONAL INFORMATION

157 calories

14.7 g fat

2 g saturated fats

9.4 g carbohydrates

1.1 g protein

0 mg cholesterol

1 mg sodium

ROASTED HONEY GLAZED CARROTS

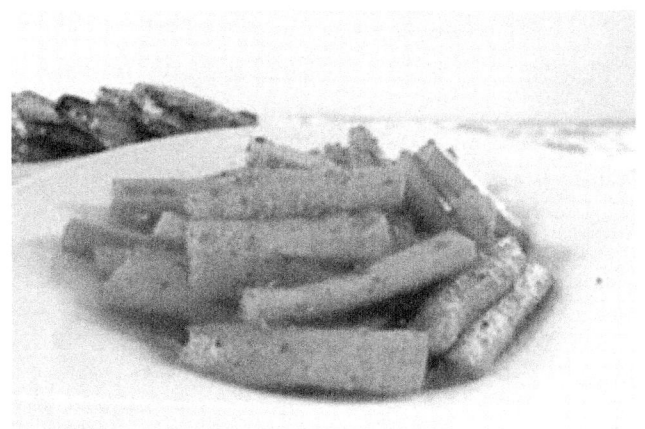

Total Prep Time: 45 Minutes

Yield: 4 servings

INGREDIENTS

- 5-6 large carrots
- Salt and pepper to taste
- 2 tablespoon Honey
- 1 tablespoon olive oil
- Chopped Parsley to garnish

INSTRUCTIONS

1. Peel the carrot and cut them into half approx. 3 inches long.
2. Add olive oil, salt, pepper, honey and carrots.
3. Toss the carrots.
4. Spread carrots on baking sheet and bake them for 400 F and for 30 mins.
5. Garnish them with parsley.
6. Serve hot.

NUTRITIONAL INFORMATION

Calorie 95

Total fat 3 g

Saturated fats 0.1 g

Sodium 344mg

Carbohydrates 16g

Sugars 4 g

Fiber 5 g

Calcium 2.5%

BLACK BEAN QUINOA SALAD

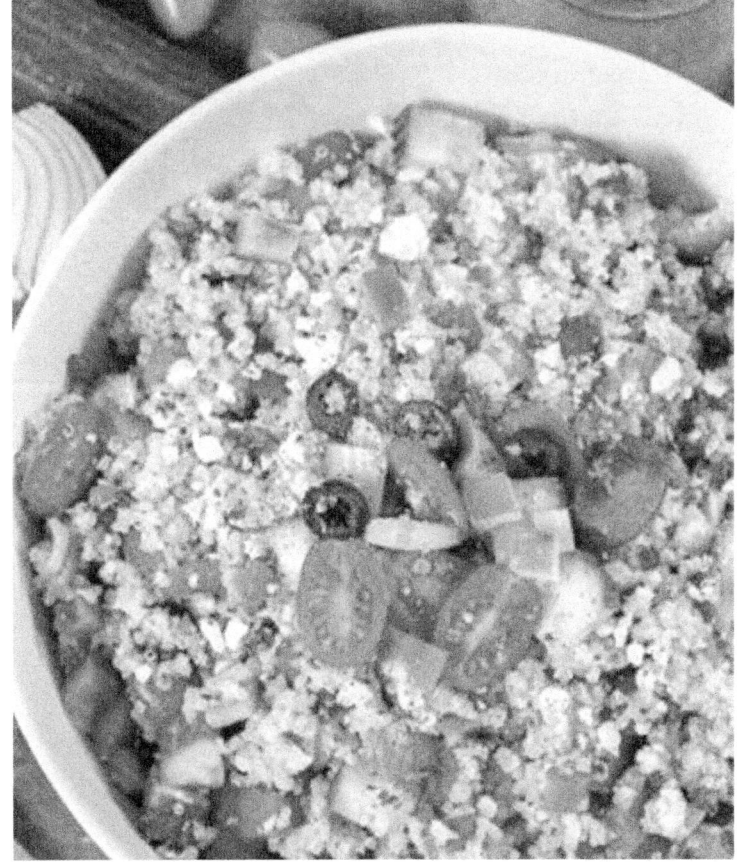

Total Prep Time: 30 Minutes

Yield: 8 servings

INGREDIENTS

- 1 cup uncooked quinoa
- 2 cups water or broth
- 2 tomatoes diced
- 1 jalapeno pepper seeded and diced
- 1 ripe avocado diced
- 1 bell pepper diced
- 1-15 oz can black beans well rinsed and drained
- 1-12 oz can corn drained
- ¼ Cup green onion diced
- 1/3 Cup cilantro chopped

DRESSING

- ¼ Cup vegetable oil
- 1 ½ Tablespoon lime juice
- 1 Teaspoon sugar
- 1 Teaspoon cumin
- ¼ Teaspoon garlic powder
- ½ Tablespoon red wine vinegar
- 1/8 Teaspoon salt
- ¼ Teaspoon pepper

INSTRUCTIONS

1. Cook your quinoa as per the package directions and let it cool.

2. To a bowl, place the quinoa and add to it the tomatoes, green onion, avocado, black beans, corn, jalapeno cilantro and bell pepper.

3. In another suitable bowl, add all the dressing ingredients slowly and let it mix well.

4. Pour your dressing over the vegetables in the bowl and toss it around to allow it to get coatd.

5. Refrigerate for some time until ready to serve.

NUTRITIONAL INFORMATION

Calories 206

Fat 11g

Saturated Fat 6g

Sodium 65mg

Carbohydrates 22g

Fiber 4g

Sugar 4g

Protein 4g

Calcium 1.9%

SIMPLE SAVORY QUINOA

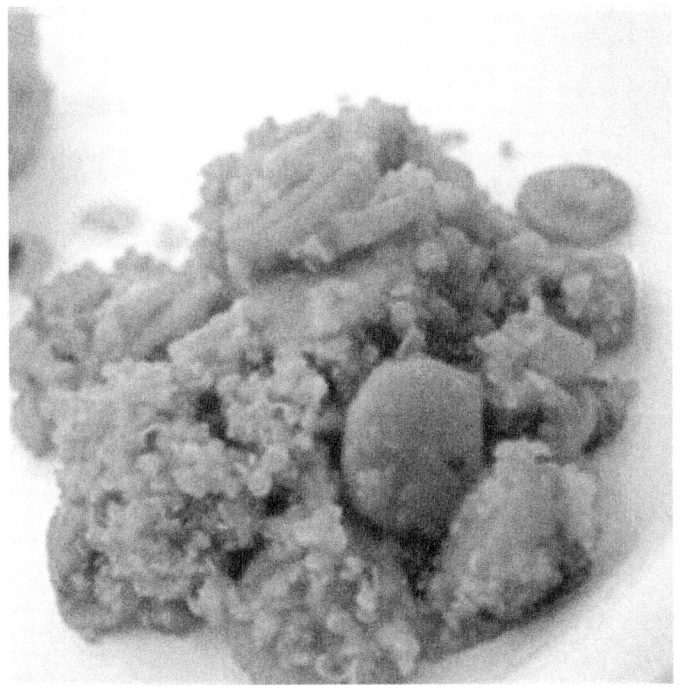

Total Prep Time: 30 Minutes

Yield: 4 servings

INGREDIENTS

- 2 tablespoons olive oil

- 1 stalk celery, finely chopped
- 2 carrots, sliced
- 1 small onion, minced
- 1 clove garlic, minced
- 1 cup vegetable stock
- 1/2 cup uncooked quinoa, rinsed
- 1/4 teaspoon dried basil
- 1 teaspoon ground turmeric
- 1 teaspoon lime juice
- salt to taste

INSTRUCTIONS

1. In an oiled and heated pan, stir in the celery, carrots, onion, and garlic.

2. Keep cooking and stirring til the onion softens and becomes translucent, this takes about 5 minutes.

3. Add the vegetable stock and stir, then add the quinoa, basil, and turmeric.

4. Allow it to a simmer, then lower the heat from medium to low and cover the pan and allow it to simmer for around 25 to 30 minutes till all the quinoa feels tender and the liquid is absorbed the.

5. Once done, stir in the lime juice, and season to taste with salt to serve.

NUTRITIONAL INFORMATION

227 calories

11.1 g fat

2 g saturated fats

27.3 g carbohydrates

6 Sugars

3 Fiber

5.2 g protein

0 mg cholesterol

195 mg sodium

5.6 % calcium

JASMINE GREEN ICE TEA

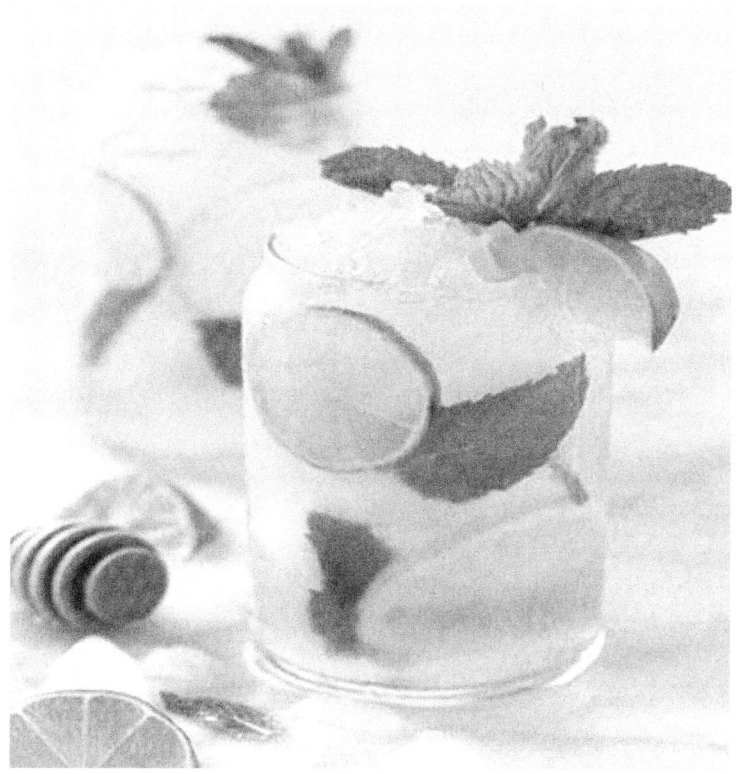

Total Prep Time: 5 Minutes

Yield: 1 serving

INGREDIENTS

- 5 tea bags, Jasmine Green Tea Bags
- 1/4 cup of lemon juice, plus 2 lemons sliced for garnish
- 5 cups of water, (2 cups boiling, plus 3 cups cold)
- 1/4 cup of honey
- 19 mint leaves

INSTRUCTIONS

1. Transfer the lime juice & lemon juice to a suitable pitcher.
2. Let 2 cups of water boil over medium heat in medium saucepan.
3. When the water becomes 170 to 185°F, add five green tea bags into the hot water.
4. Let it steep for three minutes and gently press the tea bags using a spoon against the pan to extract the tea more and more.
5. Slowly remove and throw away the tea bags from the pan.
6. Add the honey, and stir until it all dissolves.
7. Pour the tea and honey mixture into your pitcher.
8. Pour the reamining 3 cups of cold water to the pitcher and stir
9. Serve chilled green tea with ice cubes, a few lime slices, lemon slices and 3 fresh mint leaves in each glass.

NUTRITIONAL INFORMATION

Calories 46

Fat 0.01g

Saturated Fat 0.001g

Cholesterol 0mg

Sodium 5mg

Carbohydrates 13g

Fiber 3g

Sugar 3g

Protein 13g

Calcium 0.2%

BEST SUPER FOODS FOR WEIGHT LOSS

Are you struggling to reduce those extra pounds? If yes, then you will find a lot of guidance in this chapter. Reducing your weight isn't as easy as actually gaining it. However, that shouldn't discourage you. On the contrary, this should motivate you to start the journey early. Luckily, with a little help from this chapter, you'll get there sooner than expected.

Life might seem daunting right now because you are probably in the initial stages of weight loss, but trust me, it gets better. Diet is an integral aspect of weight loss. Diet doesn't mean eating less; it means eating the right kind of food that assists in weight loss.

Mechanisms for weight loss:

1. Burn more calories than you ingest
2. Ingest less calories
3. Combine both

Burning calories is not only via exercise, it can also be done via food! Yes, you can lose weight while eating, but that is only if you eat the right foods. Certain foods can raise your metabolic rate which will cause your body to burn faster.

You can ingest fewer calories by eating food that is low in carbs and fats and high in protein or fiber. We provide you with a list of food that fits all the above criteria.

You can also gain weight via hormones that are released during stress or chronic inflammation. By eating food that blocks inflammation via antioxidant activity or that induces relaxation by containing magnesium, you can curb one of the vicious circles for weight gain by a simple technique, eating the right food.

However, the best thing to do is to combine all the above strategies.

I am sure your biggest challenge is finding the right food for weight loss. Well, I have good news for you. Here's a list of foods that will help you reduce your weight.

1. Green Vegetables

The essence of weight loss includes burning more calories than you ingest. To help you with your weight loss journey, it would help to decrease your calorie intake. That might seem like it means to eat less. But then we are faced with the problem of hunger. The key is in eating food that is low in calories, that way, you can eat a voluminous amount of that type of food to get full without worrying about the number of calories you are ingesting in total.

 On top of the fact that green vegetables are packed with healthy and essential nutrients, they are also low on calories and carbohydrates. Carbs are some of the foods you should avoid if you are attempting weight loss. When you add vegetables to your diet, you don't have to reduce your intake of food. Simply eat as many green veggies as you wish without worrying about weight gain. It is carbohydrates, and food high in calories which is what causes weight gain and it's good news that vegetables are low on carbs.

Green vegetables will increase the volume of food in your stomach but at the same time keep your calorie levels in check. What's more, the high levels of fibre will help to keep you feeling full all day. Therefore, you will feel full without weight gain. They also have antioxidants which keep your immunity in check and help you burn fats.

2. Lean Beef

It is a common misconception that all meat is bad. This is not true. Even though processed meat might be unhealthy, eating unprocessed red meat will not raise the chances of suffering from diabetes or heart diseases. In fact, fresh lean beef is healthy and full of proteins and very low on fat. When buying a piece of meat, avoid the fatty pieces and opt in for the lean ones, that has more meat than fat. In fact, a lean beef cut has less than 2 grams of fat and about 55 calories.

It is also rich in proteins. The level of protein in meat helps in weight loss. Eating proteins will help you burn more calories daily as protein can be used to build muscles and muscles burn more energy. Lean beaf is low in fat and is a very healthy option for weight loss.

3. Lemon

Did you know that you can passively lose weight every day with this simple trick? Drinking lemon infused in warm water every morning on an empty stomach is an effective weight loss strategy. That is because lemon helps improve your metabolic rate.

The metabolic rate is the rate at which your body burns calories to supply your cells with energy needed for life. The higher your metabolic rate, the faster you will be burning energy and soon enough, you will be burning away the fat stores stored under your skin. When you raise your metabolic rate with drinking lemon daily, you allow your body to tap into its fat stores to burn it for energy.

You also need to drinking a lot of water for weight loss, therefore, infusing your water with lemon can help improve your health in addition to offering faster weight loss options.

4. Broccoli

A tasty variety that you can add to your weight loss diet is broccoli. This food is hands down one of the best vegetables for weight loss. This is due to its nutritious value, high fiber content and tasty appeal. It can help you to curb hunger and maintain low blood sugars, which are necessary for achieving weight loss. If you have high circulating blood sugars, some of them eventually get converted into a storage form which adds weight to your body.

Fiber is one of the essentials when it comes to weight loss. One of the easiest ways to increase your fiber intake is through eating broccoli. Fiber helps you to feel full fast so that you don't feel hungry or get hunger cravings. So, in addition to being low in carbs and low in calories, broccoli can help you eat less and therefore intake less calories to achieve a faster weight loss.

5. Strawberries

To lose weight, you need something to speed up the fat metabolism processes in your body. That is, the fat breaking processes in your body. Strawberries are one of the most suitable candidates for this job. They are a dense source of phenolic acids which support your weight loss journey because of their powerful antioxidant activity.

Not only are strawberries delicious, but they will also have a high concentration of flavonoid which prevents weight gain. Therefore, as you work on your exercise and reducing your weight, this fruit will ensure you are able to reduce your weight. They contain lots of healthy nutrients that help improve your immunity and fat metabolism such as vitamin C, calcium and magnesium.

If you are feeling hungry, a cup of strawberries can help curb the hunger with its fiber content with less than 50 calories.

Moreover, the strawberries contain anti-inflammatory agents, these agents help block the inflammatory processes which release the cortisol hormone. Cortisol released due to inflammation promotes weight gain and strawberries put a stop to the inflammation worsening.

6. Avocado

As you know, fats are a source of weight gain, an important one. However, there is a misconception, and it's important to remember that not all fats are bad. In fact, some fats are healthy, necessary and don't contribute to weight loss. These fats are monounsaturated fatty acids.

Avocados are packed with monounsaturated fatty acids which give you the fat content you need without causing you to gain weight. Moreover, they contain phytochemicals that support the fat burning metabolism and help you to lose weight. In addition, it is rich in fiber which will help you keep a healthy digestive system. A healthy digestive system is essential to have a healthy weight loss process. Moreover, the fiber will help you feel fuller faster, so you can increase your intake of avocados to feel full without worries about the calories.

Additionally, people who eat a lot of avocados have a lower BMI compared to those who don't. The combination of the fat and fiber ratio in avocados will help slim you down.

7. Beans

Beans are particularly high in fiber content. Fiber helps to reduce your appetite while at the same time promoting weight loss. Therefore, they should be your best friend if you are trying to reduce your weight. On top of that, beans also have other health benefits which include, lowering blood pressure and reducing risks of suffering from heart disease. These are the perfect easy side dish if you want to add some bulk to your dishes, or salad, for example.

8. Blueberries

One of the easiest and healthiest additions you can add to your diet is blueberries. This easy snack can help you lose weight without you noticing. The presence of anthocyanins in blueberries have been found to promote weight loss. Anthocyanins encourage your body to produce the adiponectin hormone. This hormone increases metabolism while suppressing your appetite hence causing you to take in less food which eventually results in weight loss. Adiponectin is also in charge of fat mobility and metabolism.

Inflammation also blocks the hormones that are responsible for weight loss and releases hormones that lead to weight gain such as cortisol. By taking foods rich in anti-inflammatory compounds, for instance, blueberries, you will be able to restore your weight reducing hormones and curb the production of hormones such as cortisol which lead to weight gain.

9. Yoghurt

Yoghurt is an incredible source of food for losing weight. It is tasty, can be included in many recipes and quite easy to snack on without worrying about your diet. It has probiotic bacteria which improves how your gut functions. Meaning, with a healthy gut, your body will be able to prevent leptin resistance and inflammation, both of which contribute to obesity. Leptin is also known as the satiety hormone, helping you to feel full. If you have adequate amounts of leptin circulating in your body, you can count on feeling full after eating some yogurt, although it is a relatively less bulky food.

10. Salmon

Finally, salmon is a good food when it comes to reducing your weight. It is rich in healthy unsaturated fats. These fats provide your body with a healthy fat balance without causing you to gain weight. Salmon is also rich in Omega-3 and other high-quality proteins that will help you feel satisfied while keeping watch of your calories. Moreover, it boosts your general health and helps your metabolic rate to keep burning fats. This will ensure you have the right nutrients and still manage to reduce your weight.

TOP SUPER FOOD RECIPES FOR WEIGHT LOSS

A COLOURFUL VEGETABLE PAN SHEET WITH LEMON MARINATED CHICKEN

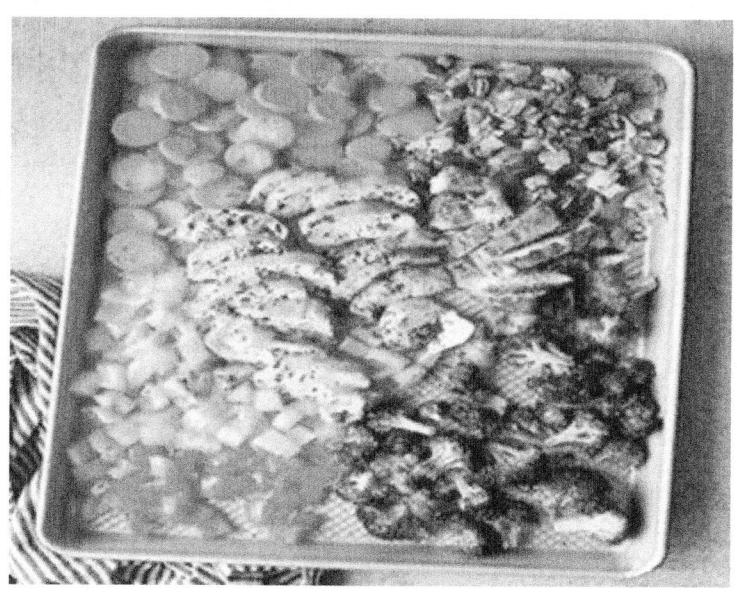

Total Prep Time: 40 minutes

Servings: 7 servings

INGREDIENTS:

- For the protein: 3 and a half Boneless Chicken Breasts

For the Marinade:

- 1 Lemon
- 2 teaspoons of Lemon Zest
- 5 tablespoons of olive oil
- 2 teaspoon of honey (optional) for sweet taste

For the Seasoning:

- teaspoons sea salt
- 1 teaspoon dried oregano
- 1 teaspoon dried thyme
- half a teaspoon black pepper
- 1 teaspoon garlic powder
- 1 teaspoon smoked paprika

For the Rainbow Vegetables

- 3/4 a cup of cherry tomatoes, cut in half
- 3/4 cup of red bell pepper, cut into 1" chunks
- 3/4 cup chopped carrots
- 3/4 orange bell pepper, cut into 1" chunks
- 3/4 yellow bell pepper, cut into 1" chunks

- 3/4 cup snap peas
- 3/4 cup broccoli florets
- 3/4 cup chopped zucchini
- 3/4 cup baby potatoes cut in half
- 3/4 cup purple baby potatoes cut in half
- 3/4 cup radishes

INSTRUCTIONS

1. Prepare the vegetables by chopping and peeling what needs to be peeled. Make sure you don't cut too big or too small pieces.
2. Preheat the oven to 400 F.
3. Start marinating the chicken breasts by adding and mixing the lemon juice and olive oil along with the honey (optional) and dip the chicken breasts in the marinade mixture. Add the lemon zests to season to the chicken breasts.
4. Add your chopped vegetables to the marinade mix and stir evenly.
5. Arrange the vegetables into your pan sheet after you grease and cover it with a baking sheet. You can arrange the vegetables according to color or size.

6. Add the remaining marinade mix from the bowl into the pan and spread it over the vegetables.

7. Add the chicken to the tray and put it in the oven for 8-10 minutes then change the chicken over to the other side and let it back in the oven.

8. If your vegetables are done, i.e. they start to look brownish and have become a lot softer, you can remove them if they are entirely cooked or scramble them if they are half baked to distribute the heat.

9. Keep the chicken for another 10 minutes and until you feel it is well cooked.

10. Divide your vegetables into servings.

11. The chicken could be cut up into smaller pieces or larger pieces to be distributed among the seven sections with the vegetables.

NUTRITIONAL INFORMATION

Calories 72

Total Fat 14g

Saturated Fat 2g

Cholesterol 99mg

Sodium 740mg

Carbohydrate 17g

Fiber 3g

Sugars 5g

Protein 33g

Calcium 10%

LOW-CALORIE EGG MUFFINS

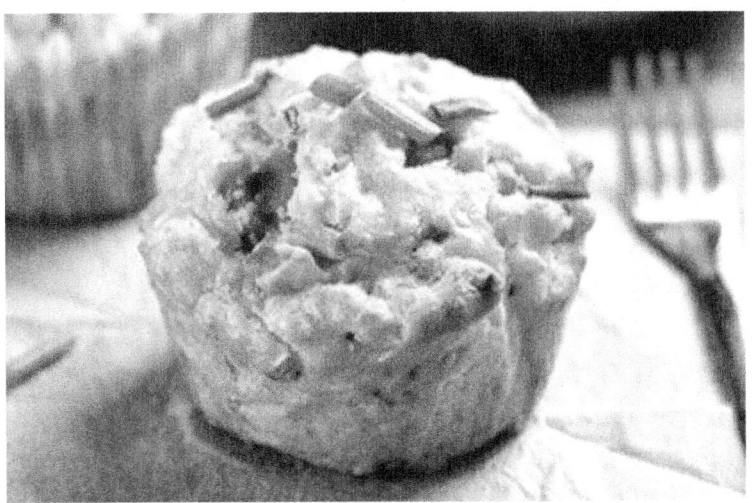

Total Prep Time: 30 minutes

Servings: 6 servings

INGREDIENTS

- 8 eggs
- 1/2 teaspoon pepper
- 1/2 teaspoon salt
- 2 cups of mixed vegetables, finely chopped small cubes such as zucchini, onion, peppers, torn spinach, mushrooms, broccoli florets

- 1 cup of shredded cheese
- 1/2 cup all-purpose flour
- 1/2 teaspoon baking powder

INSTRUCTIONS

1. Beat the eggs well then add in the salt and pepper and the vegetables of your choice.

2. There are 2 ways in which you can add the vegetables. Either add all the vegetable mix in the entire batter so that all the muffins will have the same mix or in your muffin pan, add in one or two types of vegetables to create a unique mix for each muffin for variety.

3. It is actually optional to add in the flour and baking powder the recipe does fine without them however they become a bit soggy when reheated if it is done without the flour. If you don't mind that, you will have a lower carb intake by leaving out the flour.

4. Pour the batter into the muffin pan that is layered by muffin papers or a silicone sheet and bake for 10-20 minutes until fully baked.

NUTRITIONAL INFORMATION PER SERVING

Calories 152

Fat 9 g

Saturated Fat 4 g

Cholesterol 162 mg

Sodium 265 mg

Carbohydrate 8 g

Fiber 1 g

Sugars 1 g

Protein 9 g

Calcium 3%

SOUTHWEST MIX VEGETABLE SALAD

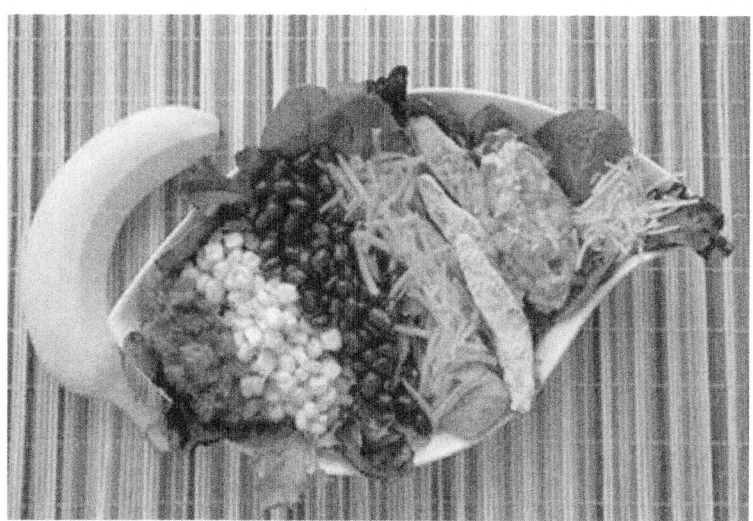

Total Prep Time: 15 minutes

Servings: 5 servings

INGREDIENTS

- 3 cups Spring mix lettuce
- 1 Tablespoon Shredded cheese
- 1/4 cup Salsa
- 3 Chicken strips
- 1/3 cup Corn

- 1 - 100 calories pack Wholly Guacamole
- 1/4 cup Black beans
- 1/4 cup shredded carrots
- 1 Banana

INSTRUCTIONS

1. You can either use canned precooked vegetables (beans and corn), or you can boil the vegetables to make sure they are cooked.
2. In a skillet, add olive oil and grill the chicken over medium heat.
3. Add all the ingredients together and mix, then add the chicken on top.

NUTRITIONAL INFORMATION

Calories 462

Fat 9 g

Saturated 2 g

Cholesterol 0.2 g

Carbohydrates 6 g

Sugar 1 g

Protein 6 g

17g of fiber

Sodium 115 mg

Calcium 12%

WHITE BEAN AND CHICKEN CHILI

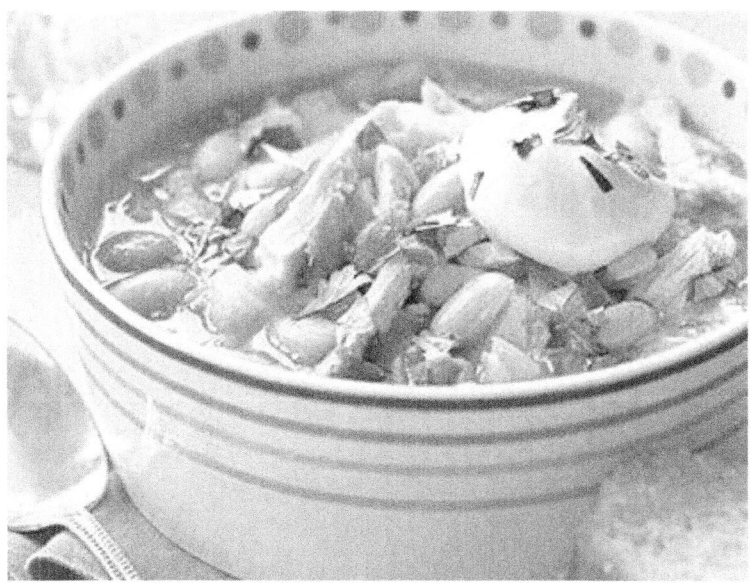

Total Prep Time: 45 minutes

Servings: 6 servings

INGREDIENTS

- 1/4 teaspoon ground cinnamon
- 4 teaspoons olive oil
- 2 pounds ground chicken
- One 14ounce can of reduced-sodium chicken broth

- 1 clove garlic, crushed with a press
- 1 medium onion, chopped
- 1 teaspoon salt
- 1 teaspoon ground cumin
- 1/2 teaspoon dried oregano
- 1/4 teaspoon ground cayenne pepper
- Two 15 ounce cans of white kidney beans (cannellini), rinsed and drained
- One 16-ounce jar mild salsa verde
- 2 tablespoons fresh cilantro leaves, for garnish

INSTRUCTION

1. Using a Dutch oven and heat one teaspoon oil on medium-high heat.
2. Add one teaspoon of salt to the chicken. Add your chicken to the Dutch oven and let it cook until the chicken is thoroughly cooked and stir frequently.
3. Remove the chicken to a medium bowl when it is done. When the chicken is cooked, put the remaining two teaspoons of oil along with the garlic and onion to the Dutch oven, and cook on medium heat while stirring every once in a while, for 5 to 6 minutes.

4. Add the cayenne pepper, cumin, oregano, cinnamon and stir for 1 minute.

5. Finally, put the broth, beans, salsa verde and the cooked browned chicken, and bring it to a boil. Reduce the heat and cover and cook the chili for 15 minutes to blend the flavors. To serve, garnish with cilantro.

NUTRITIONAL INFORMATION

Calories 350

Fat 8 g

Saturated 2 g

Cholesterol 0.1 g

Carbohydrates 4 g

Sugar 1 g

Protein 15 g

15g of fiber

Sodium 132 mg

Calcium 10.2%

CHICKEN PEA AND AVOCADO MASH SALAD

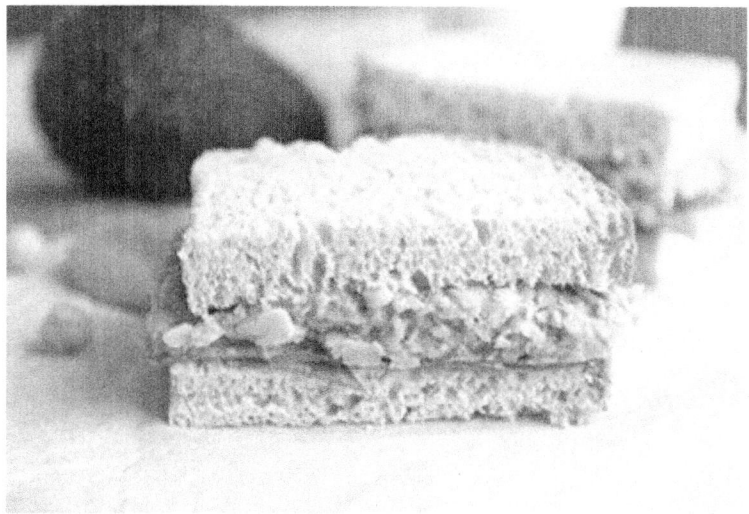

Total Prep Time: 15 minutes

Servings: 3-4 servings

INGREDIENTS

- 1/4 cup fresh cilantro, chopped
- 1 (15 ounces) can chickpeas or garbanzo beans
- 1 large ripe avocado
- Salt and pepper, to taste

- 2 tablespoons chopped green onion
- Juice from 1 lime
- Spinach leaves or any other sandwich toppings for example lettuce, tomato slices, sprouts, etc.
- Bread of your choice (I use whole wheat bread)

INSTRUCTIONS

1. Wash and drain the chickpeas.
2. Dry on a paper towel and peel of the outer skins (optional).
3. In a suitable bowl, mash the chickpeas and avocado using a fork.
4. Add to the mash the cilantro, green onion, and the lemon juice and add salt and pepper, to taste.
5. You can spread the salad on bread and top with your favorite sandwich toppings. You can top with fresh spinach leaves.

NUTRITIONAL INFORMATION

Calories 382

Fat 7 g

Saturated 1 g

Cholesterol 0.0 g

Carbohydrates 12 g

Sugar 2 g

Protein 18 g

13g of fiber

Sodium 142 mg

Calcium 8.2%

ROASTED POTATOES

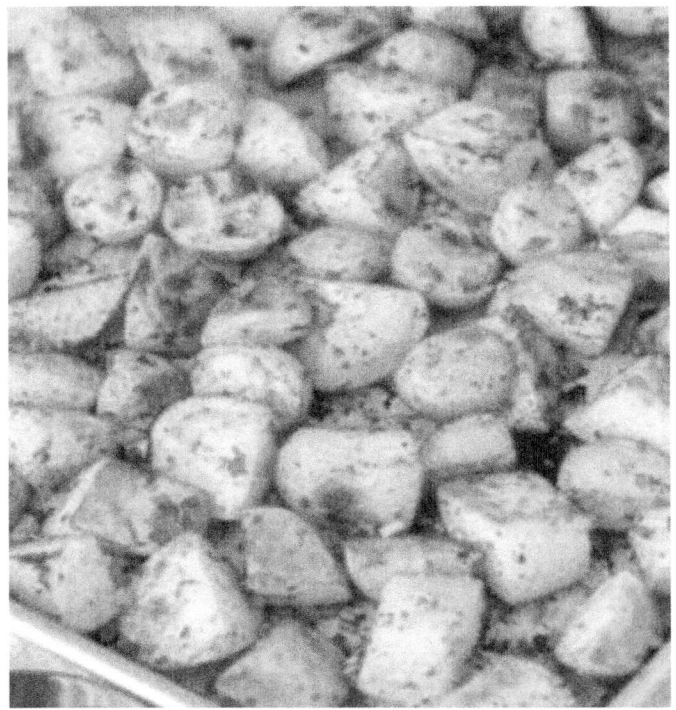

Total Prep Time: 35 minutes

Servings: 3-4 servings

INGREDIENTS

- 2 lbs red or yellow skinned potatoes

- 3 tablespoons chopped fresh herbs, for example, rosemary, parsley, thyme, basil
- 1 teaspoon garlic powder
- 2 tablespoons olive oil
- ½ Teaspoon paprika
- Add coarse salt and pepper to season

INSTRUCTIONS

1. Preheat the oven to 425 degrees.
2. Wash the potatoes well and dice them into 1" cubes.
3. (optional) If you have time, soak the potatoes in cold water for up to 1 hour then drain and dry the potatoes well.
4. On a baking sheet, place the potatoes, sprinkle olive oil, herbs and seasonings and bake for 30 minutes or until the color browns.

NUTRITION INFORMATION

Calories 147

Fat 4g

Sodium 27mg

Carbohydrates 24g

Fiber 2g

Sugar 1g

Protein 2g

Calcium 1.5%

LEMON HERB BAKED SALMON

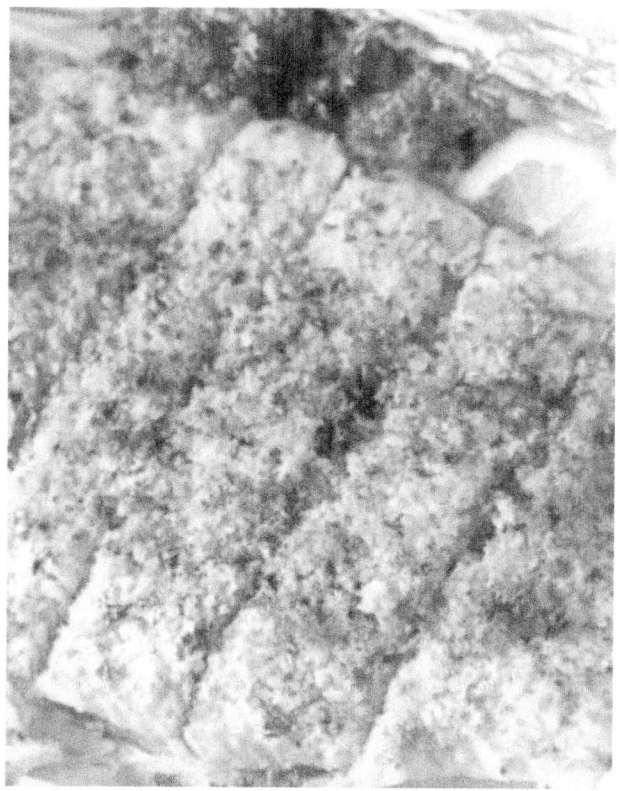

Total Prep Time: 40 minutes

Servings: 6 servings

INGREDIENTS

- 1 salmon fillet 3-4lbs
- 2 tablespoons butter melted
- 1 lemon divided use
- Salt & pepper
- Topping
- ¾ Cup Panko bread crumbs
- 3 Cloves garlic minced
- 2 tablespoons fresh parsley minced
- 1 tablespoon fresh dill minced
- zest from one lemon
- 2 tablespoons parmesan cheese shredded
- 3 tablespoons butter melted

INSTRUCTIONS

1. Preheat oven to 400 degrees.
2. Mix all ingredients in a bowl.
3. Put foil around a pan and spray with oil or cooking spray.
4. Put the salmon in the foiled pan and brush it with soft melted butter and add salt and pepper for seasoning and squeeze 1/2 of the lemon on top.

5. Sprinkle the crumb mixture on top of the salmon and bake it uncovered for 13 to 17 minutes or until you feel that the salmon flakes easily and feels or looks cooked.

NUTRITION INFORMATION

Calories 377

Fat 20g

Saturated Fat 6g

Cholesterol 128mg

Sodium 212mg

Carbohydrates 5g

Sugar 1 g

Protein 40g

Calcium 5.7%

SPLASH SUMMER CHICKEN SALAD

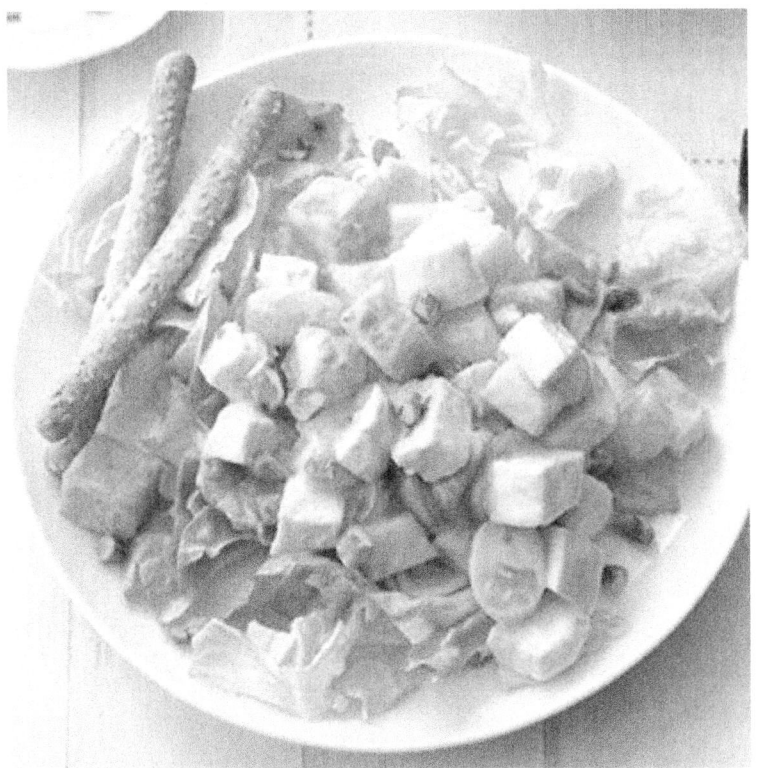

Total Prep Time: 20 minutes

Servings: 4 servings

INGREDIENTS

- 1/2 cup plain yoghurt

- 1/2 teaspoon grated lime zest
- 4-1/2 teaspoons brown sugar
- 2 cups cubed cooked chicken breast
- 1/4 cup chopped pistachios, toasted
- 1 tablespoon lime juice
- 1/4 teaspoon salt
- 1 cup chopped watermelon, seeds removed
- 1 cup green grapes, halved
- 1 cup diced peeled mango
- 4 cups of lettuce

INSTRUCTIONS

1. Mix the yoghurt, lime juice and zest, brown sugar and the salt.
2. Add the cooked chicken then add the chopped fruits.
3. Top with lettuce and the pistachio.

NUTRITIONAL INFORMATION

Calories 263

Fat 8g

Saturated fat 2g

Cholesterol 0 mg

Sodium 248 mg

Carbohydrate 27 g

Sugars 22g

Fiber 3 g

Protein 24 g

Calcium 8.3 %

FROZEN GREEK YOGHURT

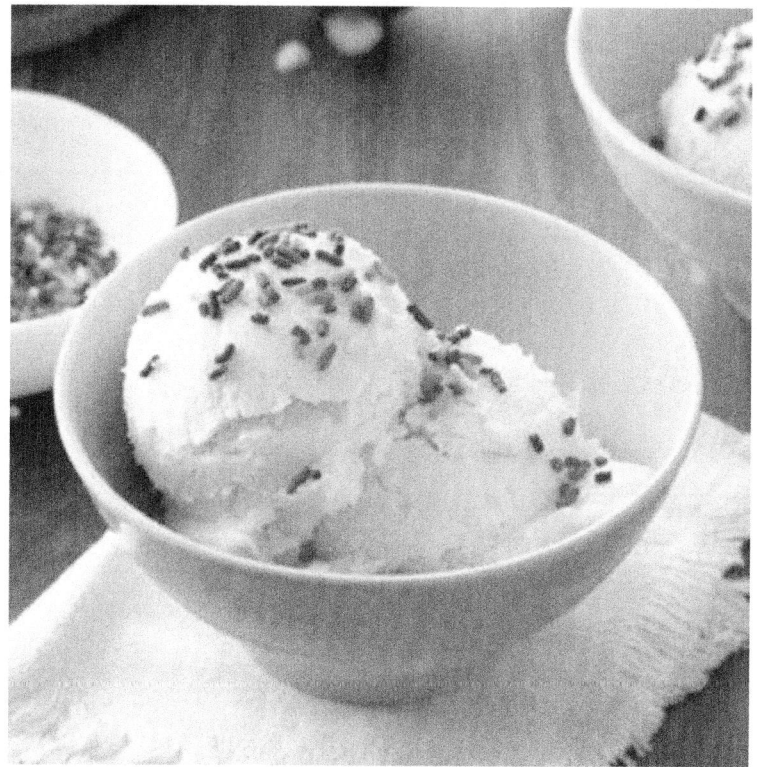

Total Prep Time: 7 hours

Servings: 2-4 servings

INGREDIENTS

- 3 cups reduced-fat plain Greek yoghurt

- 3/4 cup sugar
- 1 teaspoon unflavored gelatin
- tablespoon lemon juice
- 1/2 teaspoons vanilla extract
- 1 tablespoon cold water

INSTRUCTIONS

10. Use a strainer and line it with layers of cheese cloth or coffee filter and put it over a bowel.

11. Place yoghurt in prepared strainer; cover yoghurt with sides of cheesecloth.

12. Refrigerate 2-4 hours.

13. Remove yoghurt from cheesecloth to a bowl; discard strained liquid.

14. Add sugar and vanilla to yoghurt and stir until the sugar is dissolved.

15. In a microwave-safe bowl add cold water and the lemon juice; then sprinkle it with gelatin and let it stand for 1 minute.

16. Put the mixture in the Microwave in the high setting for thirty seconds, frequently stir until the gelatin is completely melted. Add the mixture to the yoghurt.

17. Cover the mixture it and put it in the fridge to refrigerate until cold for around 40 minutes.

18. Pour yoghurt mixture into the cylinder of ice cream freezer; freeze according to the manufacturer's directions.

19. Transfer frozen yoghurt to a freezer friendly container and freeze for 2-4 hours or until you get consistency firm enough to scoop like ice cream.

NUTRITIONAL INFORMATION

Calories 224

Fat 3 g

Saturated fat 2 g

Cholesterol 7mg

Sodium 57 mg

Carbohydrate 36

Sugars 36 g

Fiber 0

Protein 13 g

EASY KALE SALAD WITH FRESH LEMON DRESSING

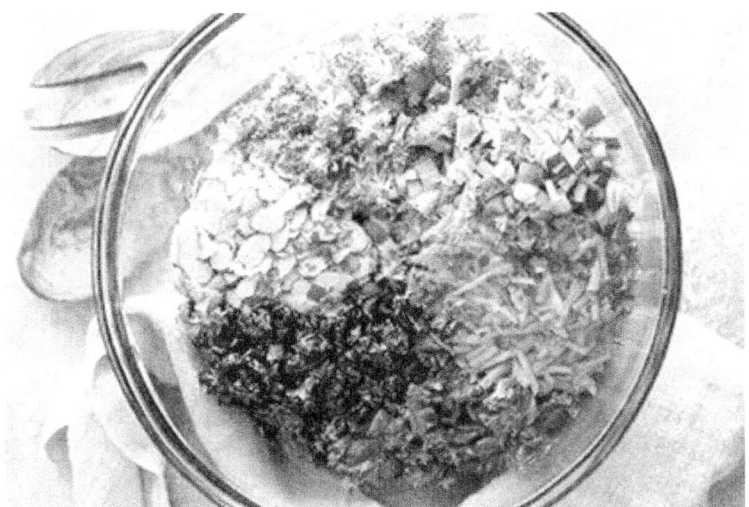

Total Prep Time: 20 minutes

Servings: 4 servings

INGREDIENTS

- 5 cups chopped kale
- 1-2 tsp olive oil
- 1/2 cup sliced almonds
- 1/8 tsp salt

- 2 cups chopped broccoli
- 1/4-1/2 cup shredded carrots
- 1/2 cup cheese optional
- ¼ Cup diced red onion
- ¼ Cup sunflower seeds
- ¼ Cup cranberries
- Lemon Dressing
- ¼ Cup olive oil
- 2 tbsp fresh lemon juice
- 2 Teaspoons red wine vinegar
- 1 Teaspoon Dijon mustard
- 1 clove garlic minced
- ½ Teaspoon dried oregano
- ¼ Teaspoon salt
- 1/8 Teaspoon ground black pepper
- 1 Teaspoon honey or sugar adjust + add to taste

INSTRUCTIONS

1. To make the dressing by adding the ingredients above in a covered mason jar then shaking well to thicken.

2. Put a kale leaf in the prepped dressing and add sweetener, salt, and pepper to taste.

3. Sprinkle some olive oil and a pinch of salt to your chopped kale.

4. Massage the leaves with your fingers till the leaves start to soften and darken.

5. In a large bowl, stir in the massaged kale, almonds, broccoli, cheese, carrots, onion, sunflower seeds, cranberries.

6. Shake the dressing then pour about 1/3 of the dressing over the salad. You can add more as preferred.

NUTRITIONAL INFORMATION

Calories 333

Fat 26g

Saturated Fat 3g

Cholesterol 0

Sodium 316mg

Carbohydrates 19g

Fiber 5g

Sugar 4g

Protein 9g

Calcium 19.2%

CONCLUSION

I hope you have enjoyed reading this book and have been introduced to new and exciting recipes. Super foods are a great way to enhance your health and protect your body and your organs against chronic illnesses and boost your energy levels. With the recipes in this book, each powered with at least 2 super foods, you can heal your body while having fun cooking for you and your family. Don't be afraid to try new recipes or modify any of the recipes in the book according to your needs.

Food is the traditional ultimate healer and first line of prevention against disease, by maintaining a good health. Make sure you are adding super foods to your diet daily.

Happy Cooking!

Printed in Great Britain
by Amazon

79791709R00153